FULL GAS FOREVER

FULL GAS = a rider pushing themselves to their maximum abilities.

FOREVER = for all future time; for always.

FULL GAS FOREVER

A 40+ CYCLIST'S GUIDE TO RIDING FASTER AND FURTHER

ED CLANCY AND
LEXIE WILLIAMSON

BLOOMSBURY SPORT
LONDON · OXFORD · NEW YORK · NEW DELHI · SYDNEY

BLOOMSBURY SPORT
Bloomsbury Publishing Plc
50 Bedford Square, London, WC1B 3DP, UK
Bloomsbury Publishing Ireland Limited,
29 Earlsfort Terrace, Dublin 2, D02 AY28, Ireland

BLOOMSBURY, BLOOMSBURY SPORT and the Diana logo are trademarks of
Bloomsbury Publishing Plc

First published in Great Britain 2025

Copyright © Ed Clancy and Lexie Williamson, 2025
Photography © Tony Blake, 2025 with the exception of the following; pp. 154, 165 and
177 © Getty Images

Ed Clancy and Lexie Williamson have asserted their right under the Copyright,
Designs and Patents Act, 1988, to be identified as Author of this work

For legal purposes the Acknowledgements on p.187
constitute an extension of this copyright page

All rights reserved. No part of this publication may be: i) reproduced or transmitted in
any form, electronic or mechanical, including photocopying, recording or by means
of any information storage or retrieval system without prior permission in writing from
the publishers; or ii) used or reproduced in any way for the training, development or
operation of artificial intelligence (AI) technologies, including generative AI technologies.
The rights holders expressly reserve this publication from the text and data mining
exception as per Article 4(3) of the Digital Single Market Directive (EU) 2019/790

Bloomsbury Publishing Plc does not have any control over, or responsibility for, any third-
party websites referred to or in this book. All internet addresses given in this book were
correct at the time of going to press. The author and publisher regret any inconvenience
caused if addresses have changed or sites have ceased to exist, but can accept no
responsibility for any such changes

Every reasonable effort has been made to trace copyright holders of material reproduced
in this book, but if any have been inadvertently overlooked the publishers would be glad
to hear from them.

A catalogue record for this book is available from the British Library

Library of Congress Cataloguing-in-Publication data has been applied for

ISBN: PB: 978-1-399-42020-4; ePUB: 978-1-399-42023-5; ePDF: 978-1-399-42024-2

2 4 6 8 10 9 7 5 3 1

Typeset in Trade Gothic Next LT Pro

Design by Emil Dacanay and Sian Rance for D.R. ink
Printed and bound in China by C&C Offset Printing Co., Ltd.

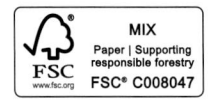

To find out more about our authors and books visit www.bloomsbury.com
and sign up for our newsletters. For product safety related questions contact
productsafety@bloomsbury.com

Note: While every effort has been made to ensure that the content of this book is as
technically accurate and as sound as possible, neither the author nor the publishers can
accept responsibility for any injury or loss sustained as a result of the use of this material.

CONTENTS

INTRODUCTION, ED CLANCY — 6
INTRODUCTION, LEXIE WILLIAMSON — 8

1 THE MIDLIFE CYCLIST — 12
2 BIKES AND BITS — 18
3 STRENGTH TRAINING — 26
4 CORE STRENGTH — 42
5 MINIMISING RESISTANCE — 56
6 FLEXIBILITY — 62
7 NIGGLES — 76
8 DOES MENTAL PERFORMANCE MATTER? — 84
9 TRAINING BASICS — 92
10 CYCLING TECHNIQUE — 102
11 TRAINING SPECIFICS — 108
12 HYDRATION — 116
13 NUTRITION — 124
14 RECOVERY — 132
15 SLEEP — 138
16 HORMONES — 146
17 GOING OFF-ROAD — 152
18 INDOOR TRAINING — 162
19 RACING — 168
20 SPORTIVES, GRAN FONDOS AND ÉTAPES — 176

EPILOGUE:
   ED CLANCY — 182
   LEXIE WILLIAMSON — 185
REFERENCES — 186
BIBLIOGRAPHY — 186
ACKNOWLEDGEMENTS — 187
INDEX — 190

INTRODUCTION, ED CLANCY

I RIDE MY BIKE NOW for the same reason I did as a kid and have always done: I love it. Some people I meet think that after a 20-year career in cycling – winning world championships, breaking world records and picking up three Olympic golds – I might have left my bike locked up in the garage forever once I retired. Nothing could be further from the truth. I still love being out on my bike.

Those hours that I spent on the rollers or going round and round a small track at the velodrome or getting soaked through riding in the driving North of England rain haven't diminished the thrill. I get such a kick out of it, whether it's gritting my teeth and grinding out every pedal turn on a mountain climb, concentrating on staying vertical on a gnarly, muddy descent in the woods, experiencing the adrenaline rush in a sprint for the finish line or cruising along chatting in the bunch.

Now, as I approach my 40s, I realise there are certain inevitable biological changes that could affect my enjoyment of being out on the bike. I've been warned. Bones feel creaky, muscles ache and energy is more quickly sapped. As a professional rider for 20 years who has crashed regularly, trained until I dropped and gone through illness, none of these will be new. The only difference will be experiencing them as a middle-aged guy and all that entails.

I'm lucky enough to still be involved with cycling at many different levels and I know that age is no barrier to not only enjoying being on a bike, but to riding at speed. I've attended and ridden in club rides, criterium races, mass-participation sportives and even online races on Zwift, where the over-40s are incredibly well represented and are often among the top riders. Cycling is one of the most suitable and achievable sports for middle-aged men and women, with age having only a minimal effect on performing to high levels.

INTRODUCTION

I believe that training as a cyclist is often overcomplicated. It is just about increasing stamina and power. Whatever your age, there is nothing stopping you improving those elements with simple training programmes. It is also about understanding that fitness is only part of cycling as a sport; there are a host of vital components, such as technique, roadcraft and mental attitude, that can be refined to aid performance. These are not areas confined to the young and can even compensate for any diminishing physical powers.

The Team GB sports psychologist, Dr Steve Peters, once sat me down and said, 'The facts of life are that the goalposts move, there's no guarantees, and life is unfair.' He wasn't being negative. He meant that you need to accept those things, adapt, prepare and move on. The same is true for mature cyclists. If you are in control of your expectations and limitations, there is no ceiling to what you can achieve.

In my own rides, on the various sportives and events I attend and in my role as Active Travel Commissioner for South Yorkshire, I encounter cyclists of all ages. So often, it is those in their middle years and older who seem to get the most out of the sport. Their attitude, ability and sheer enjoyment in being out on their bikes is inspiring and living proof that we can get fitter and faster even as the years advance. I hope this book gives encouragement, direction and guidance for those aiming to join them.

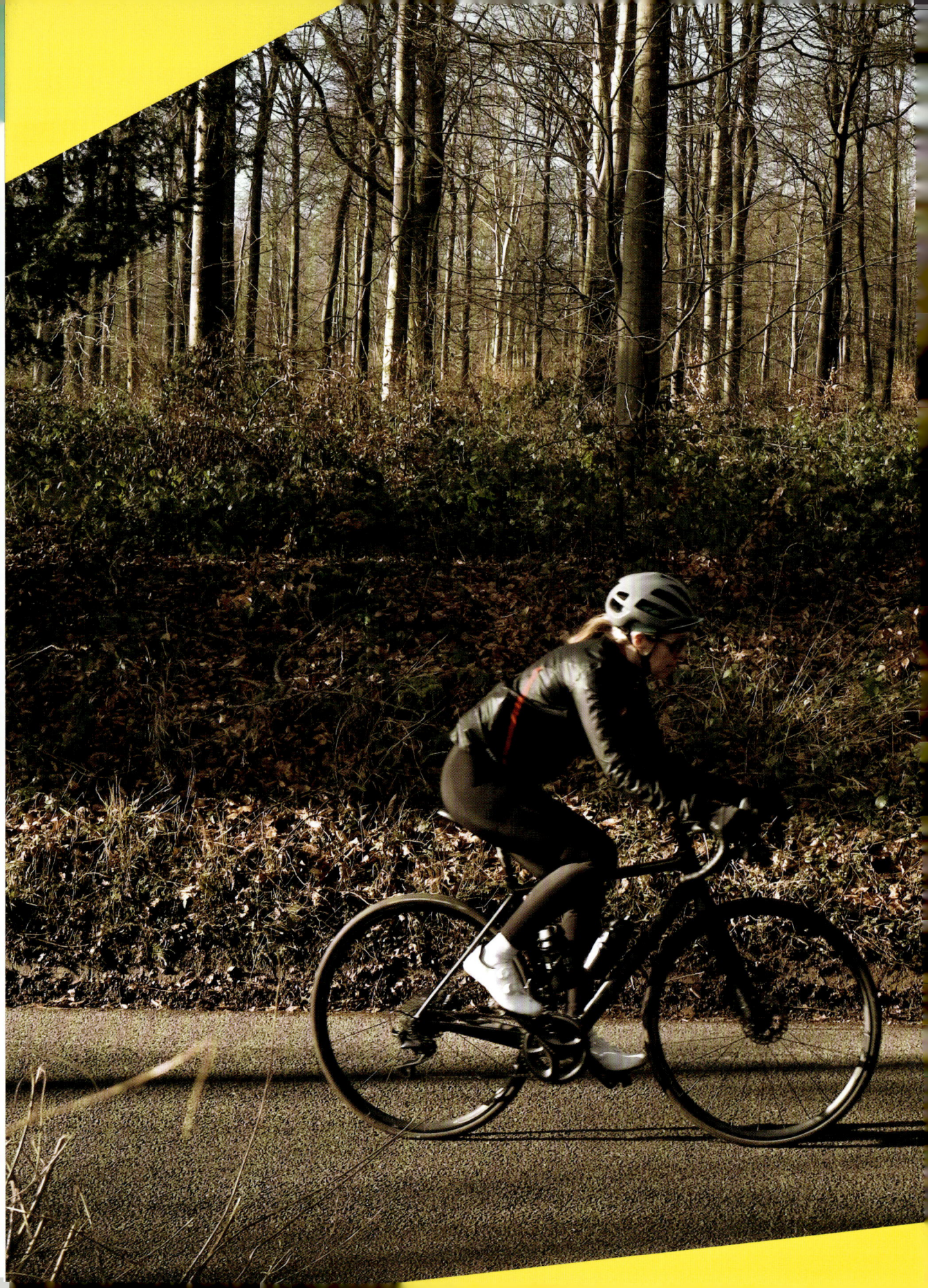

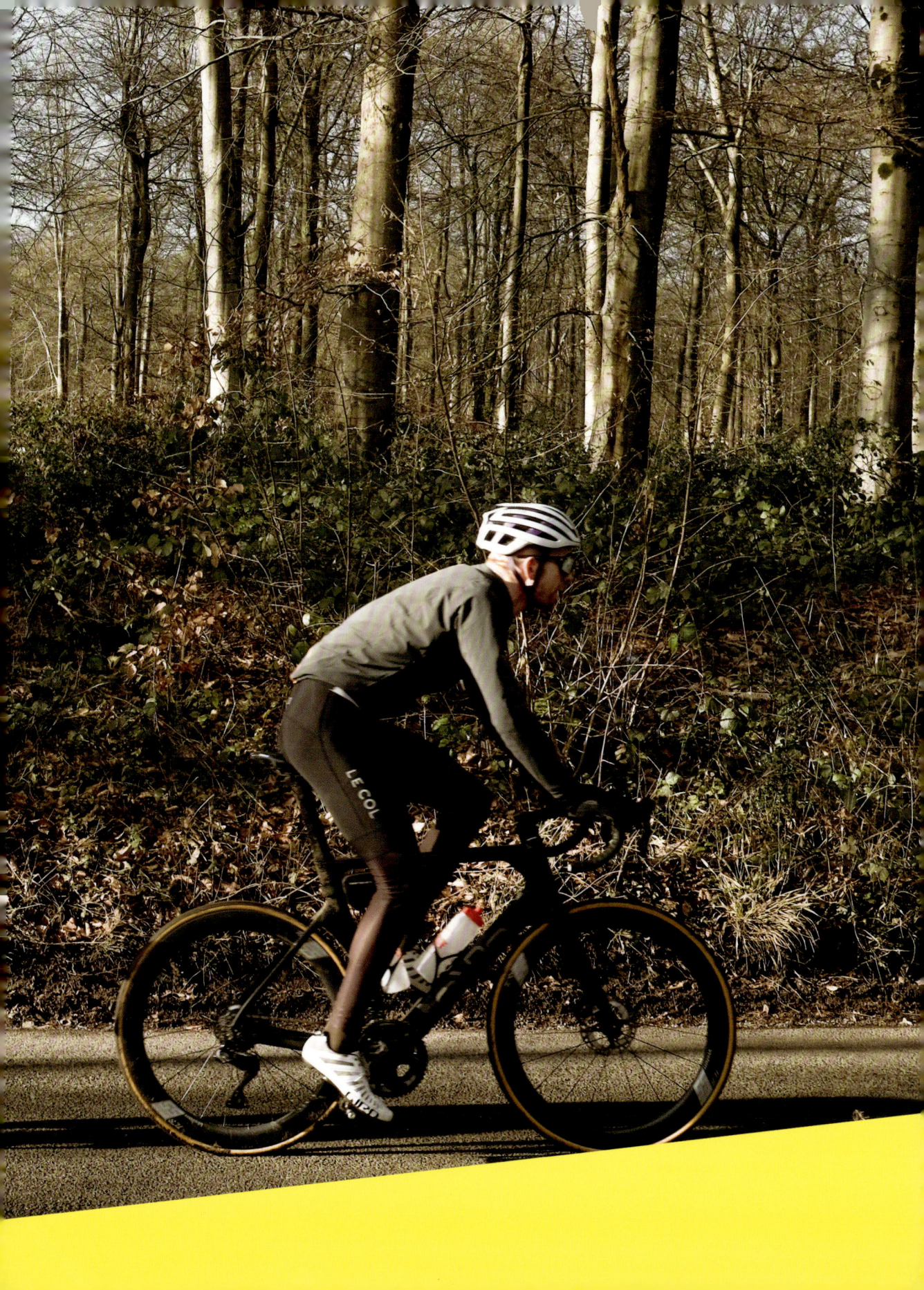

THE MIDLIFE CYCLIST

Can you be a cyclist in middle age? It's a redundant question really. How can you not be a cyclist in middle age is a much better challenge. It's the best possible exercise you can be doing as you wave goodbye to your youth. It's great for your mental state, sociability and general health, and – to get to the point of this book – there is nothing stopping you improving your performance even as the years tick over.

Generation X were the first age group to realise that you didn't have to hang up your bib shorts at the first sign of a grey hair. That you could still push yourself to be a better athlete and you wouldn't crash and burn just because you felt breathless and your heart beat a little faster. The only thing that might hurt were the hilarious 'MAMIL!' jibes from passing motorists – and that was water off a Gore-Tex rain jacket. Nowadays, thanks to those two-wheeled pioneers, it's perfectly unremarkable to see mature cyclists participating in everything from local rides, clubs, races and competitions to training camps and sportives. Older riders are welcomed with open arms and often they are present in sufficient numbers to ride or race in specific groups.

When is midlife? Few of us think of ourselves as old in our 40s. We've still got it; we can keep going and put out some serious watts when required. But as the period when ageing in the body begins to take effect, and when many women feel the effects of the perimenopause or the menopause itself, it's a fair starting point. For the general population, from the 30s onwards, we see muscle mass decrease around 3–8 per cent every decade and VO_2 max (heart and lung efficiency) takes a 10 per cent dip in the same period. In your 40s you start to lose bone mineral density at a similar rate.

Cycling is the ideal sport to take on any such decline. It is the form of exercise that is easiest on the body. There is little impact and the rotational movement puts minimal stress on many of the joints. You are therefore able to build both strength and stamina without causing undue damage to your body. While at the younger end of midlife it can help stave off age-related decreases in cardiovascular fitness and muscle mass, in older people it helps to mitigate the losses. Some scientific research has also revealed there is a link between strong legs and a fit brain, which may help with other effects of ageing.

At this point a much requoted maxim from Dr Kenneth Cooper, a pioneer of the use of aerobic exercise to maintain and improve health, is useful: 'We don't stop exercising because we get old – we get old because we stop exercising.' So, if you are already thinking that you might as well get the slippers out and ease back in your comfy armchair for the twilight years, stop right there. These diminishing powers aren't set in stone; they can be countered and ameliorated. Cyclists – and, to be fair, other kinds of athletes too – aren't the general population. This isn't the time to ease off, but to power on. The over-40s are performing to high levels in a number of sports, and scientists and coaches have realised that age does not have to restrict performance, as long as the training targets those areas that may be affected most by the ageing process.

Training hints for older cyclists

Train progressively – The body does not stop adapting to training load as you get older. With small increases in time or intensity, it continues to develop. This means that to go faster or further, your training sessions will need to get more difficult over time.

- **Build the base** – Cycling is an endurance sport. If you are going to reverse that VO_2 max decline that comes with age, you will have to do the aerobic base work with some regular long, easy rides.

Some scientific research has also revealed there is a link between strong legs and a fit brain.

There is absolutely nothing stopping you being a faster and better cyclist.

- **Core strength** – Your legs might be doing the lion's share of the work, but a strong torso provides stability, power and efficiency. Override the natural deterioration of core muscle tissue with exercises that strengthen the abs, hip flexors, pelvic floor and other muscles.
- **Get stronger** – You might prefer to be out on your bike, but find time to build strength training into your week if you want your muscles and bones to age well. Using weights will increase bone density, tendon quality and strength, and improve almost every area of your cycling fitness.
- **Power up** – Make use of high-intensity interval training (HIIT) to increase muscle strength and endurance. Combined with your endurance training, it will improve both power output and oxygen uptake.
- **Train smarter** – You may have more time on your hands now than when you were younger, but there is no need to fill it with training. Your body might or might not require longer to recover than it used to, but overtraining is more likely to cause injury. So, choose quality over quantity every time and know when enough is enough.

It is difficult to understate the level to which you can perform in these midlife years if you have the necessary commitment. True, it is rare to see a participant in professional or elite races aged over 40, but many ride competitively against younger cyclists in organised races and the standard of Masters racing is deeply impressive.

As a mature athlete, you have much more going for you than you might think. Look at VO_2 max, an accepted measurement of an athlete's ability to perform well in an endurance event. Despite the ageing effect, it is relatively easy to increase your VO_2 max (depending on your starting point, of course) through regular training. Many of the over-50s I ride with who train regularly are within the top 1 per cent in terms of VO_2 max in their age group.

The next advantage carries a big generalisation alert, but it is worth mentioning. Older people sometimes have less frantic and chaotic lifestyles. They are able to make time for training despite working, family and social commitments. They have a more measured and less madly competitive attitude. With reduced peer pressure and expectations, their mental resilience is greater, and they are able to be honest about their ability and fitness. It is also quite possible that they not only have more time on their hands, but are also less constrained by a lack of disposable income.

Technology also gives you a helping hand. In your training there are a variety of apps and programmes that provide valuable guidance and information, while pretty accurate power meters and other performance-monitoring cycling computers enable you to keep track of your progress. Bike technology is changing fast too – tyre tech, wheels, electronic gears, disc brakes and more make the bike faster without you having to do anything more than shell out for equipment.

Best of all, remember that cycling faster and longer is not just about fitness. Improvements you can make to your nutrition, recovery, bike set-up, roadcraft and bike-handling skills are not restricted by age. You have to smile when the strongest, fittest young bucks on a sportive struggle to shake off a canny, leech-like oldster!

There is absolutely nothing stopping you being a faster and better cyclist. However, it won't happen without paying attention to the ageing process. There is no point thinking you have the body of a 25-year-old. You will need to be focused and structure your training around new challenges as you get older.

Beating the ageing process

- **Stay on form** – The ageing body can be unforgiving, so don't give it a chance to trip you up. No making-do or cheating. Set up all your bikes correctly – that goes for your turbo or rollers as well as any outdoor bikes you have. When exercising or stretching, don't rush the process. Make sure that your posture is correct, that you follow the proscribed technique and don't overextend your legs or arms.
- **Be alert to pain** – Those days of riding through it are gone. Whether you are on the bike or exercising, if it hurts it is not a good sign. Your ability to repair tissue is reduced with age, so react sensibly to avoid any long-term injury. There's plenty of gain to be had without pain.
- **Be bendy** – A combination of ageing effects, from collagen reduction to dehydrated discs, can cause stiff joints. This can affect your bike position and comfort when riding, and can leave you doubled up at the end of a ride. Fortunately, a programme of yoga- and Pilates-based exercises can really help to keep the body flexible.
- **Watch the waistline** – You may be burning off the calories, but you still have to pay attention to your diet. The long-held idea that people's metabolic rate decreases in middle age has largely been debunked (scientists now believe that happens after the age of 60), but hormonal changes in men and women do make weight control more difficult. So, avoid faddish or extreme dieting and eat sensibly according to your training and riding requirements.
- **Sleep more** – While older adults don't necessarily need more sleep than younger people, sleep quality declines as we age. High-quality sleep is the time when the body replenishes its energy levels, helps the production of oestrogen and testosterone, and releases human growth hormone (HGH), which helps build muscle, burn fat and stimulate tissue growth. Getting more sleep will offer you the best possible chance of giving your body the right preparation.

FULL GAS FOREVER

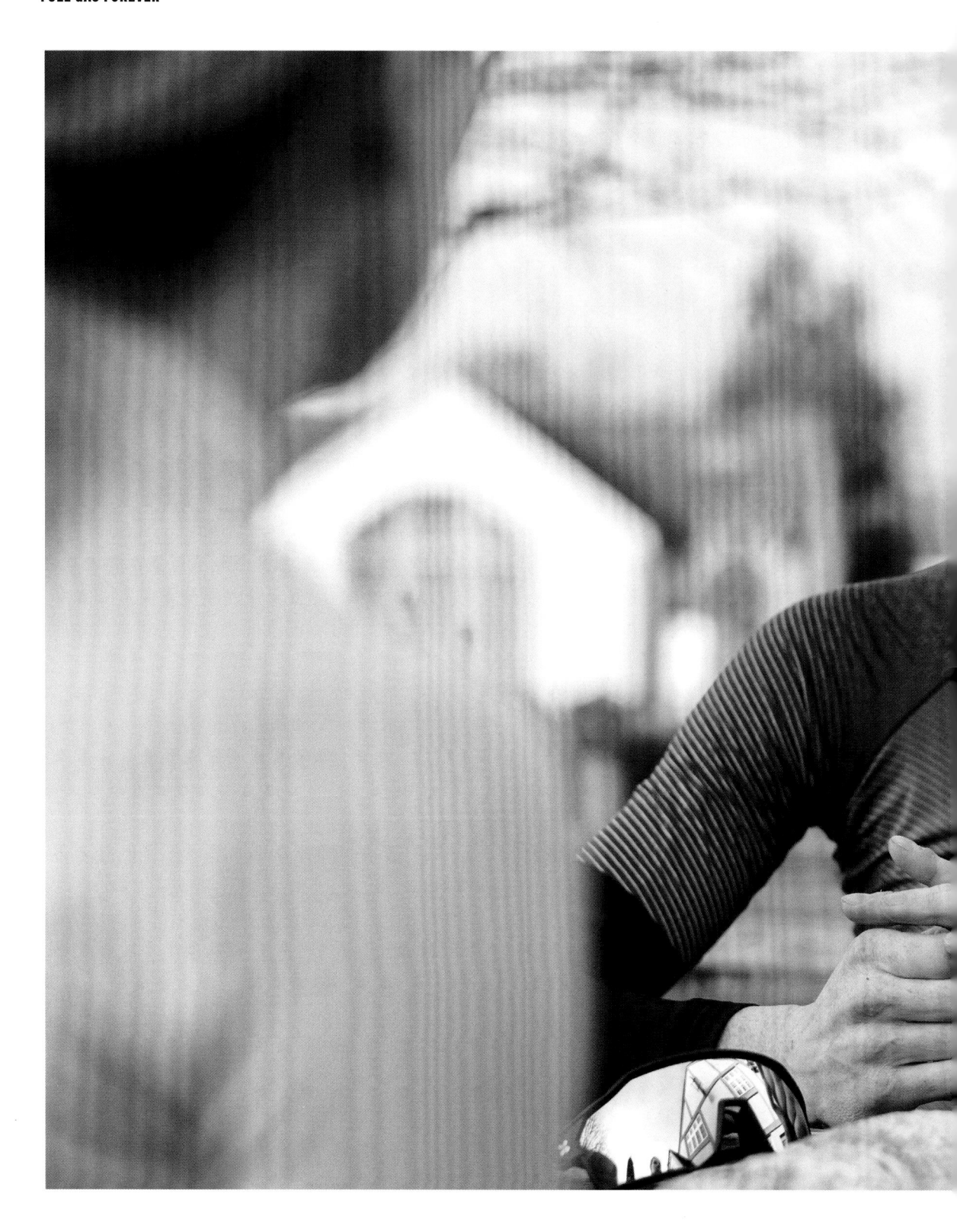

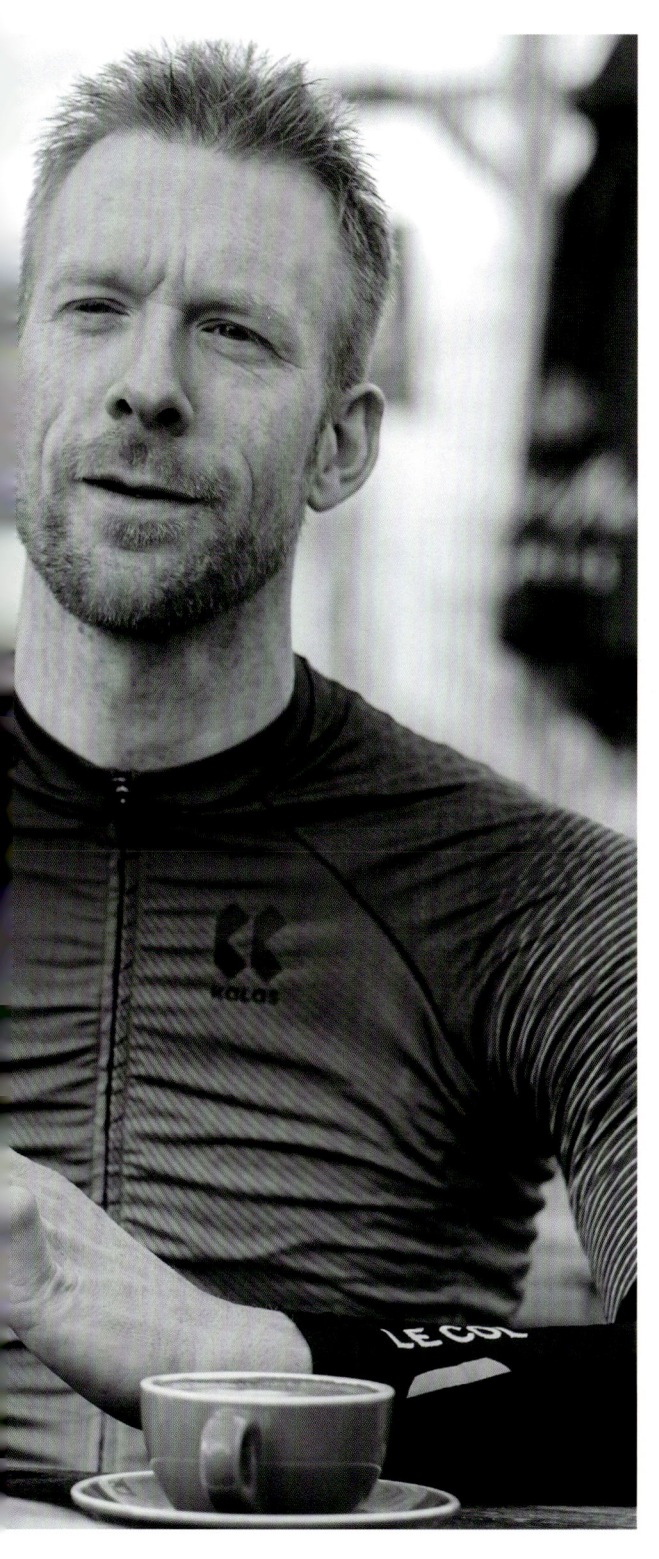

Fuel your ride and recovery

Getting the correct nutrition to support your riding and your recovery is essential as you get older and your body is less resilient to stress. Eating optimally entails giving yourself enough energy to fuel your performance and sufficient nutrients to aid your recovery after the ride or training session. Basically, that equates to a balanced diet with an emphasis on carbohydrates before and during endurance events and protein after. Older cyclists should pay greater heed to hydration as they have less body water, lose more water when they urinate and are thought to have a less sensitive perception of thirst.

As Dylan Thomas almost wrote: do not ride gentle into that final kilo. Middle age does not need to be the time to ease off the pedals. Indeed, there are many reasons, as you'll discover in the following pages, why it is a great period of your life to go full gas. As a generation, we have defied science, embraced taking fitness and performance to new heights, and shown at all levels that performance and enjoyment on a bike has nothing to do with ageing. It is a revolution that has only just begun. If you want to push yourself, there is nothing stopping you. If you just want to have fun on two wheels, then more power to you. And if you want to go faster, go for it!

BIKES AND BITS

Whether it is pure speed, climbing, endurance or technical manoeuvring, the precision engineering of even modestly priced bikes and accessories can ensure a rider's performance matches their efforts.

Your bike won't go fast on its own, but it can help. A lighter bike can make a huge difference in climbs, while on the flat as much as a quarter of the aerodynamic drag (air resistance) can be contributed by the bike itself. That is why the cutting edge of bike technology is in super-light components or aerodynamic frames, wheels and bars.

If you are happy to spend around £2000 ($2500), you will find a bike that will comfortably get you round a sportive. If you are set to race anything up to national level you will be looking more at £3000 ($3725). After that the benefits per pound become marginal. You can spend a grand or more just to save 1kg (2.2lb). Twelve-speed cassettes, special ball bearings or super tyres can make a difference, but you need to be at a level where that is worth the outlay.

Effective cycling isn't just about going fast, though. Climbing, bike handling and sheer endurance are an integral part of many cycling disciplines. So, choosing a bike should be about enabling you to ride, climb or manoeuvre in the most effective way possible. That means comfort is often as or more important than shaving a few seconds off your sprint time. You could buy a top-of-the-range time trial (TT) bike, but it would be little use if you are climbing mountains most of the day.

Brakes

The ability to brake underpins much of your confidence in your riding. Whether you are descending, riding in groups, in traffic or avoiding potholes and unpredictable obstacles, how quickly you can get yourself out of trouble is paramount. You need to be able to slow down or stop quickly regardless of anyone else's actions.

So, your brakes need to work well and be within comfortable reach at any time. Braking is a skill that needs practising. With well-maintained brakes, stopping quickly is no problem; it's what happens next that is the issue. Taking flight over the handlebars is easy and can result in serious injury, while wet and dry surfaces create their own problems. You should know how to finesse and modulate your brakes and your weight transfer – especially at the front, where you need to ease the front brake rather than snatching at it.

For a century, rim brakes were the traditional braking system on most bikes. If looked after, with pads regularly replaced, they did the job in dry conditions and you ran the risk when it was wet. For a decade, though, there has been little advance in rim brakes, with research and development focused instead on disc brakes. Originally the choice of mountain bike riders, over the last five years or so these have become standard on road bikes too and are available at a range of price points. Disc brakes are a no-brainer. Once heavier in comparison with rim brakes, the weight difference is now negligible. They generate a lot more stopping power with more sensitive lever control, work consistently across all weather conditions and wheel material, and require virtually zero regular maintenance, even self-adjusting to compensate when pads wear down.

Saddle

The saddle is the next most important part of the bike. Saddle choice is a personal thing; there is no right or wrong – it depends on our shapes and sizes, riding style and flexibility. It's just a case of finding the right one for you: one that is comfortable and prevents numbness, chafing or pain. Most good retailers offer a sale and return policy on saddles, as they understand that trial and error is part of the process.

The position of the two sit bones (which support the body when sitting down) is key to comfort and not putting pressure on soft tissue between them is vital to avoid numbness. Sit bones vary a lot from person to person so it is impossible to be very specific, and gender, riding style and discipline are important, too. Endurance riders and mountain bikers often seek the comfort of longer curved saddles, while racers tend to go

Choosing a bike should be about enabling you to ride, climb or manoeuvre in the most effective way possible.

for the shorter, narrower models. Personally, I like a split nose saddle that has a gap running down the centre of the front half. These completely take the pressure off the private parts, so they offer a more comfortable ride as well as providing stability in a forward, nose-down racing position. They take a little getting used to, but I'd say it is worth the trouble.

Split nose saddles are also a solution for many women riders, for whom saddle comfort – the one non-unisex feature on a bike – has long been an issue. Women generally have wider hips and sit bones than men, so they are more comfortable on wider saddles. Of course, shapes and sizes vary, and finding a suitable saddle can be a more difficult task for women than it is for men. Women may also suffer more from saddle discomfort as they go through the perimenopause and menopause due to genitourinary issues.

The shape of the saddle is everything. The level of padding, whether it is 2mm (0.08in) or 10mm (0.4in), isn't really important if the saddle is set up right. On the track, I've ridden on saddles made of carbon fibre. They had absolutely no padding, but, having been set up right, I felt comfortable all day.

Wheels

The choice of wheel can make a real difference, too. Here again, riding style and discipline should influence your choice of wheel material, rim depth and width. For a decade now the trend in wheel size in all disciplines of cycling has been for wider wheel rims. On mountain bikes it means wider tyres, which help with handling and grip. For road riders mainly riding on the flat, the increased aerodynamic profile of a wide rim more than balances the effect of the extra weight. Wheel rim depth follows a similar line in drag advantage over weight. Deeper rims are usually stiffer, transmit more power and are more aerodynamic, but shallower rims offer better control and are less subject to buffeting by crosswinds. The choice of material is a now familiar story. Carbon-fibre wheels are usually lighter, more aerodynamic and stiffer. They are close to a must-have if you are racing at a reasonably high level but can cost as much as your bike. For everyone else, high-end alloy wheels are less expensive and can do almost as good a job.

Tyres

It bugs me that compared to motorsport, where making tyres is almost a dark art, cycling lags far behind the curve in science, research and innovation. A £140 ($175) motorbike back tyre can have five different compounds, varying from a grippy super-soft edge to a durable hard-wearing rubber in the centre. Mountain bike tyres can incorporate three compounds, but road bikes remain steadfastly single compound.

Nevertheless, as the one part of the bike in contact with the ground, tyres are worth splashing out on. Cheap tyres can feel really draggy on the road and be prone to punctures, whereas the best ones roll fast as well as gripping well in the wet and dry. I was once in a team where all the riders used the same brand. When it was wet, corners were very difficult and we all crashed far too often. When we eventually switched manufacturers, we couldn't stop winning even when it rained.

A decent tyre can make a world of difference. It is difficult to work out what's best, though. There are few detailed tests assessing grip, compound or puncture resistance available in cycling magazines. My best advice is to discover what other cyclists use, find a brand you like and stick with it.

Tubeless tyres, where the tyre itself forms an airtight seal with the wheel rim, are really popular now. You pump the tyre up, add a small amount of sealant, and the tyre and rim form a perfect lock so air does not escape. In my experience they work unbelievably well on mountain bike tyres with thicker rubber and lower pressure. Many gravel riders have also converted, but the roadies are not wholly convinced. They are lighter than tubes, have a decreased rolling resistance and they don't blow, only losing air slowly if they puncture, so at least you have a tyre to ride home on even if it is a little soft. However, the technology is not quite there yet. With higher pressure and thin rubber, they are not as effective against punctures, and are messy and difficult to change or install, so many riders end up taking a spare tube with them anyway.

Setting the pressure in your tube is a fine balance between rolling resistance, the flexing of the tyre in contact with the ground, grip, bike stability and puncture resistance. These variants all work against each other so finding the right pressure is a subjective and tricky business, and is also affected by your weight and the terrain. For off-roaders, begin around 20psi for the front wheel and 22psi for the rear and take it from there. Traditionally, road riders went high, 120psi or more, but the use of wider tyres has brought this down to 90psi or lower.

Handlebars

One of the three major contact points, along with the saddle and pedals, handlebars are crucial to bike handling and your riding position. The major priority is to have the bars that best serve the discipline you ride. Mountain bikers will look

> *My best advice is to discover what other cyclists use, find a brand you like and stick with it.*

to have flat bars for maximum handling, leverage and balance; road riders generally have drop handlebars, which offer aerodynamic positioning and comfort through a variety of hand positions. Most drops these days have a compact shape and bend at a more acute angle than traditional bars, to give a shorter and easier reach for the rider. An alternative, which some might appreciate, is an anatomic bar, shaped to maintain the aero profile, but providing a more comfortable position for less flexible riders. Flared bars, which are wider on the drops than at the hoods, are generally preferred by gravel riders, as they provide a degree of both position and handling advantages, but increasingly they are being seen on road bikes, too.

In my opinion, if you are looking to go racing, bikes come with handlebars that are too wide. Most bikes are sold with handlebar widths that match the frame size, from 40cm (15.8in)-wide bars on small bikes to 44cm (17.3in)-wide ones on large bikes. It isn't something you should immediately worry about; the first thing to look for is a comfortable fit with bars that match your shoulder width. However, swapping to a narrower bar can be an easy aerodynamic win, as there is very little trade-off between comfort and power production.

In terms of material, the options are aluminium or carbon fibre. Carbon-fibre bars are generally fitted on high-end bikes. They are easily moulded into comfortable and aero shapes, are strong enough to pass safety tests and weigh 50g (1.8oz) or more less than aluminium bars. However, many pro and elite riders still plump for the cheaper aluminium option. They like the extra stiffness and the fact that they are less likely to be damaged in

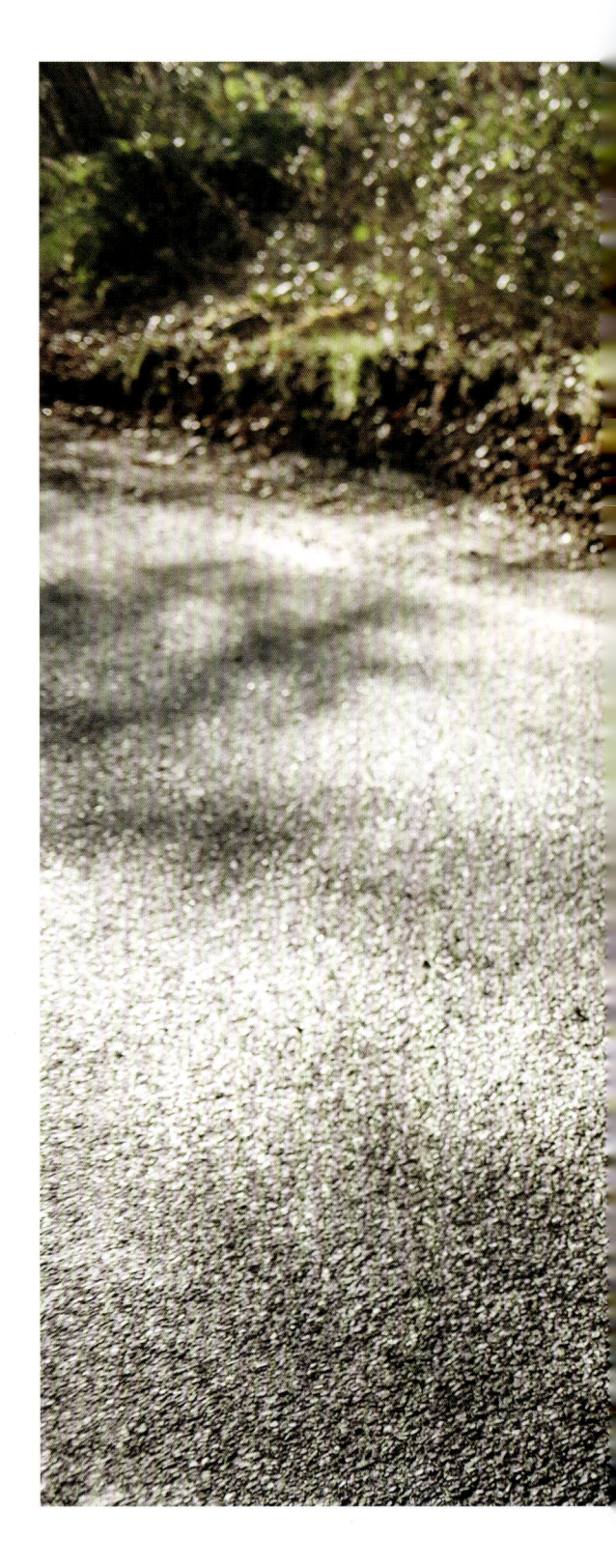

BIKES AND BITS

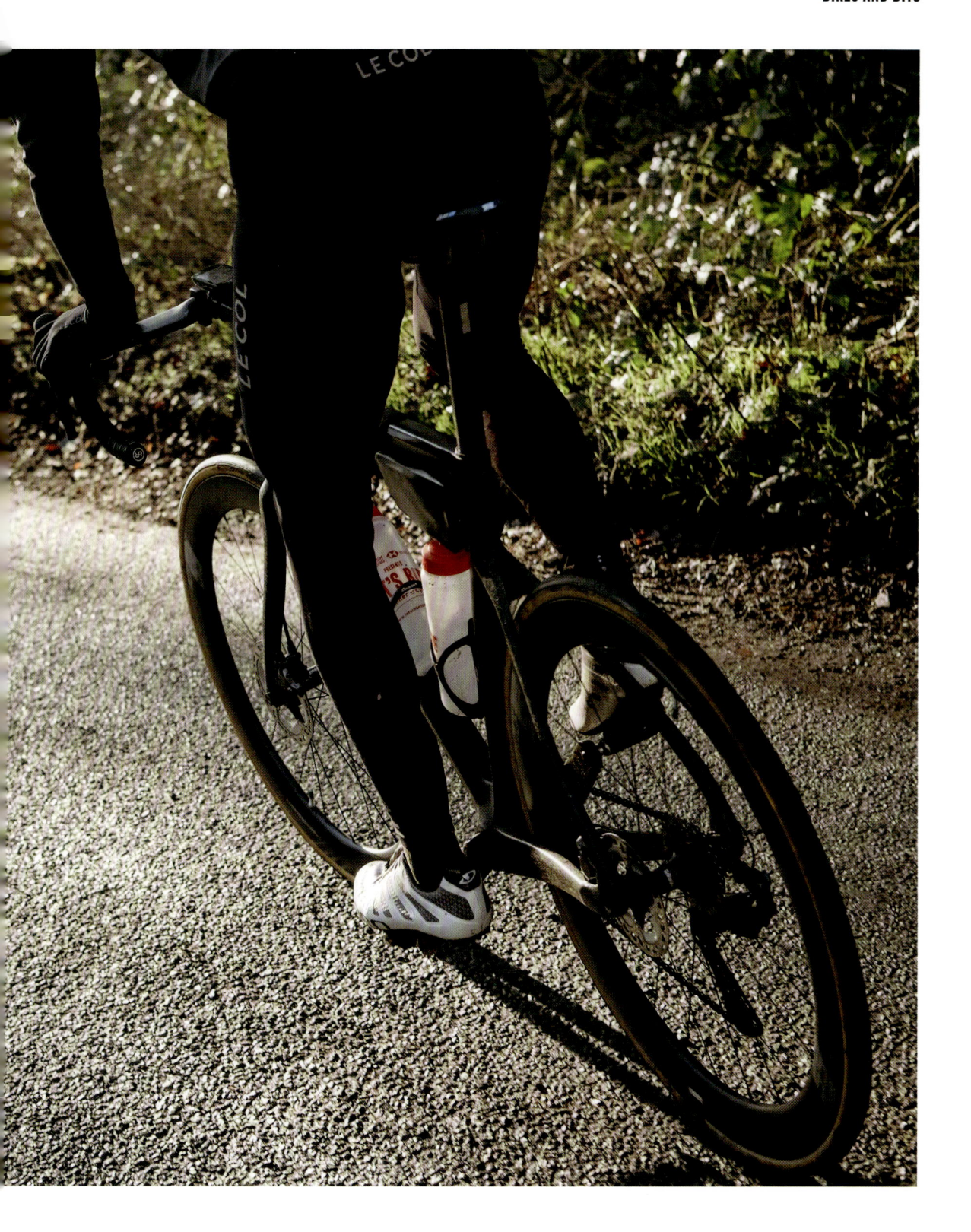

a crash or a knock. It's your choice, but unless you are really looking for marginal gains in weight (and some style points), it's probably worth passing on the carbon-fibre integrated bar and stem units.

Pedals

While on mountain bikes there is still some debate over clipless pedals with cleats versus flat pedals. On the road clipless pedals have long since won any argument. They are comfortable and fast, transmitting power efficiently at the most effective point. If you haven't worn them before, they can take a little getting used to – and we've all had the embarrassing keel-over at traffic lights. Most people adapt really quickly, though, and the perseverance pays off with more than 25 per cent more power being generated.

At the lower price range, pedals are multi-discipline, but MTB and gravel racing pedals have a wider platform than road pedals. It's worth investing around £100 ($125) in decent pedals and the same in shoes, with only marginal gains to be made with more expensive items.

Gears

The days when electronic gears were untrustworthy are long gone. Even at a cost of around £1000 ($1250), they're a bit of a no-brainer now technology has ironed out the mech disasters and solved annoying battery issues in the rain, and they now add just 100–200g (3.5–7oz) to the bike. While cable gears were subject to stretched and worn cables, electronic gears give you reliable gear changes every time, and changing is almost effortless, so there's no fumbling with numb fingers in the cold. They are cableless, easy to set up and have smart features to communicate with GPS systems and apps. The batteries are easily charged and long-lasting. I charge mine once a month and could ride a week-long stage race on a single charge.

Frame

What kind of riding you intend on doing will define your frame choice, as the geometry (shape) and materials are designed for specific functions. Endurance bikes aim to reduce fatigue and are built to absorb vibration and bumps; racing and time trial bikes are all about the aerodynamics. The geometry is geared to an aggressive riding position, and they have integrated components and aero tubes. Bikes more suited to climbing have a more upright position with more weight over the rear wheel. That said, Welsh cyclist Geraint Thomas rides a whole Grand Tour on the same bike (apart from the time trial).

Putting the heavier and more expensive steel and titanium options aside, the choice of material again comes down to carbon fibre or alloy. The expensive carbon-fibre option offers a light and stiff frame that can be moulded easily to provide aerodynamic gains, while a higher-end (but still cheaper) aluminium frame can often offer similar advantages.

Maintenance

These days, I buy my own bikes and look after them myself. If I ride my road bike in the sun and it's relatively clean when I finish, I don't touch it. I'll do four or five rides like that in Spain or in the UK if it doesn't rain. Then I'll hose it down, spray it with bike cleaner, get some degreaser on the chain, leave it for two or three minutes, then hose it off. Cleaning it gives you the chance to spot any problems, such as a piece of glass on the tyre, the rear brake pads looking worn or a rear brake hose leaking hydraulic fluid,

Oil your chain. When I'm on a sportive, I can sometimes hear someone's chain grating away, dry-thrashing with every pedal stroke. Honestly, it hurts my soul; I can feel the sprockets in the chain wearing away exponentially fast. After at least every 10 rides, get the old oil off, clean the chain and re-oil it. If you use decent cleaning products and lubricate the drive chain well then most of the components can last many thousands of miles.

That said, some parts will just wear out. The tyres (the rear first) and brake pads, whether they are disc or rim, need replacing as soon as they're worn. A chain checker for under £10 ($12.5) can tell you how worn your sprockets and chain rings are, and you can just use your ears to listen out for grinding bearings, cranks rattling in the bottom bracket or a grating headset.

> *Oil your chain. When I'm on a sportive, I can sometimes hear someone's chain grating away, dry-thrashing with every pedal stroke. Honestly, it hurts my soul.*

STRENGTH TRAINING

3

Lexie Williamson

We'd all choose the open road over the gym, but if there's a recurring theme in this book it is lift, lift, lift, even if it's only your bodyweight. Evidence is overwhelming that resistance training will combat the age-related decline in muscle mass, boost your watts and prevent injury. Hey, it might even give you the quads of a 20-year-old. But it's easy to overdo it and ruin your riding legs. Let us ease you in with a gentle, bike-specific approach.

Midlife cyclists' strength training

Let's just jump straight in with four damn good reasons why you should strength train:

1. It prevents 'brittle' (and easily fractured) bones

Cycling, unlike running, is a non-impact sport, so it doesn't maintain bone density. This puts cyclists who only ride at the risk of fracturing bones when they crash. Cyclists have been found to have shockingly low bone mineral density (BMD). Indeed, studies have shown them to have the same, or even lower, BMD as sedentary people.

We need, therefore, to load our bones with running or weight training. As Phil Cavell says in his book *The Midlife Cyclist*, 'The road to becoming a great cyclist in middle age and beyond may well involve doing less cycling in favour of other activities.' It's all about longevity; sacrifice a session now and ride blissfully into middle age and beyond.

2. It could give you the muscle power of a 20-year-old

This is probably the only argument you're reading ... but another depressing result of getting older is that we lose muscle mass as we age and this rate accelerates over the age of 60. This is called sarcopenia. Before you lose all hope, targeted weight training will cause the muscle fibres that you have left to hypertrophy or increase in size. According to Cavell, this will result in 'function and power closer to someone in their mid-20s' — and who doesn't want that!

3. It helps support those poor overworked quads
Cyclists tend to overuse their quads and neglect the strongest muscles in the legs, the glutes (buttocks/buns/derrière/tush). Exercises like squats and lunges will build the gluteus maximus and gluteus medius at the side of the hips. These muscles add a lot of power and stability to each pedal stroke.

4. It makes you more durable
Resistance training will reinforce weaker areas of the body, which can start complaining as the miles wear on, such as the lower back, and space around the shoulder blades and the back of the neck. It will also support joints such as the knees, which is particularly useful for long rides when fatigue sets in. In a nutshell, improved lower body strength in particular will help you tolerate the high training loads that are the bread and butter of the serious midlife cyclist.

How to start strength training — and how not to

My attempts at adopting strength training have been pretty disastrous. Bombarded by images of cyclists performing deadlifts on social media, I headed to the gym to give it a go and piled on the weights. Result? A 'tweaked' lower back that put me out of riding action for weeks. A few months later I hired a personal trainer to nail my technique, but suffered with the dreaded delayed onset muscle soreness (DOMS), to the detriment of my riding.

It turns out that I was doing it (like a lot of things) all wrong.

It was time to wheel in an expert who, as a former pro triathlete turned cyclist, understood that my priority was riding. He assured me that it *is* possible to strength train and keep your legs fresh.

Meet endurance strength specialist Chris Panayiotou, who has a system for gym newbie cyclists to start resistance training that he promises won't negatively impact their performance on the bike. 'A good strength programme will try to minimise DOMS so it doesn't have a detrimental effect on your cycling,' he says. You might get a little DOMS on your first or second session, but when volume and load are managed effectively it will be less and less each time. It's also not about 'absolute' strength (the amount you can lift) but 'relative' strength (being strong in comparison to your bodyweight).

These are Chris's three pieces of advice for cyclists who are new to the gym:

FULL GAS FOREVER

> **'Say what?' The lingo to pass off as a gym pro**
>
> **Reps** – A single execution of an exercise.
> **Sets** – A group of reps.
> **Supercompensation** – The physiological adaptation to training load resulting in performance improvements.
> **Intensity** – This refers to the amount of weight lifted. For example, 'low intensity' involves lifting a relatively light weight or doing only a few reps with a heavier weight, while 'high intensity' involves using heavy weights or doing a high number of reps with a lighter weight.
>
> *Source: Road Cycling Academy*

If you don't move well and then load your body with heavy weights, there is a much greater risk of injury.

1) Hone your movement patterns

'When we start strength training we're not looking at particular muscle groups but instead movement patterns,' says Panayiotou. It is essential for athletes, regardless of their strength level, to move well. He advocates practising movement patterns that involve multiple joints trained together, or 'compound' movements. 'Instead of isolating single groups we can get the biggest bang for our buck with compound movements and maximise our training time,' he says.

2) Start without weights

Perfecting movement patterns brings us on to the second related theme: start strength training just using your bodyweight. Why? Because if you don't move well and then load your body with heavy weights, there is a much greater risk of injury. 'Think about deadlifting at your maximum level; the movement pattern often breaks down, leading to a loss of technique and huge increase in injury risk.' He adds, 'Always chase the [are you ready for another acronym?] MED or "minimal effective dose". This is the smallest amount of strength training needed to elicit an improvement in performance.' The beauty of using bodyweight is you don't actually need a gym at all. You can do it anywhere.

3) 'Slow and steady wins the race'

Yes, it's not the cycling way, but doing too much too soon is a recipe for sore legs and injury. Just do a session lasting under an hour once or twice a week. This session can replace one of your rides. Tough, I know, but you will reap the rewards.

How-to: bodyweight strength training for cyclists

Chris Panayiotou has created a four-week bodyweight strength training routine for cyclists that revolves around four movement patterns: **push**, **pull**, **anterior chain** (muscles at the front of the body) and **posterior chain** (muscles at the back of the body).

Each section has several exercises, which become progressively harder. Remember to keep it simple, be safe and progress slowly.

PUSH

1 WALL PRESS

Start standing at arm's length away from a wall with your feet shoulder-width apart. Place your hands on the wall at shoulder height, slightly wider than shoulder-width apart. Keep your body in a straight line from head to heels. Engage your core muscles. Bend your elbows and lower your chest towards the wall while keeping your body straight. Push against the wall to straighten your arms and return to the starting position.

Do 8–10 reps in weeks 1 and 2, increasing to 10–12 reps in weeks 3 and 4.

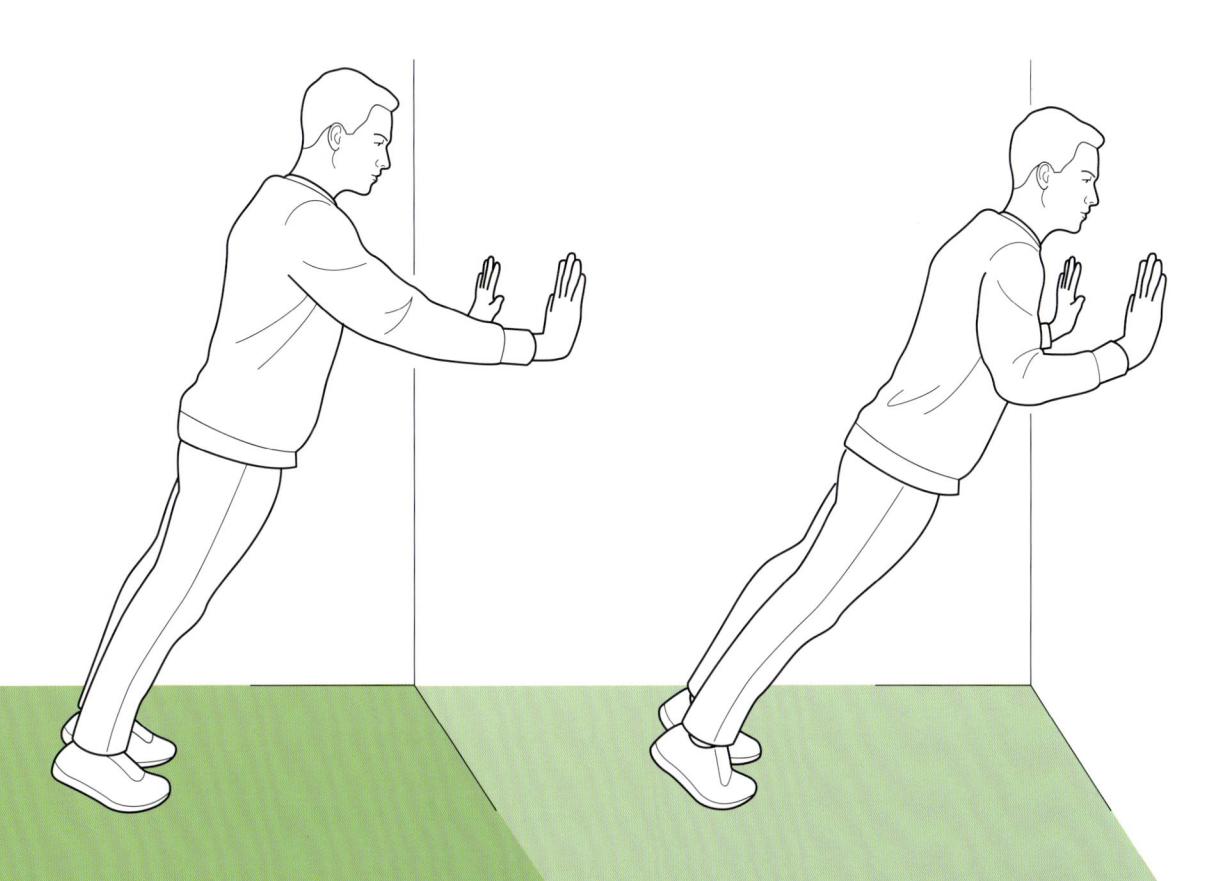

2 KNEELING PUSH-UP PLANK

Start on all fours with your hands directly under your shoulders, knees bent and feet off the floor. From here, walk your hands forward until the body forms a kneeling push-up position. Engage your tummy muscles and glutes, and hold.

Do 2 x 10–15-second holds with five seconds' rest between, working towards a 30-second static hold with no rest. Once you can complete this, try the kneeling hand release push-up.

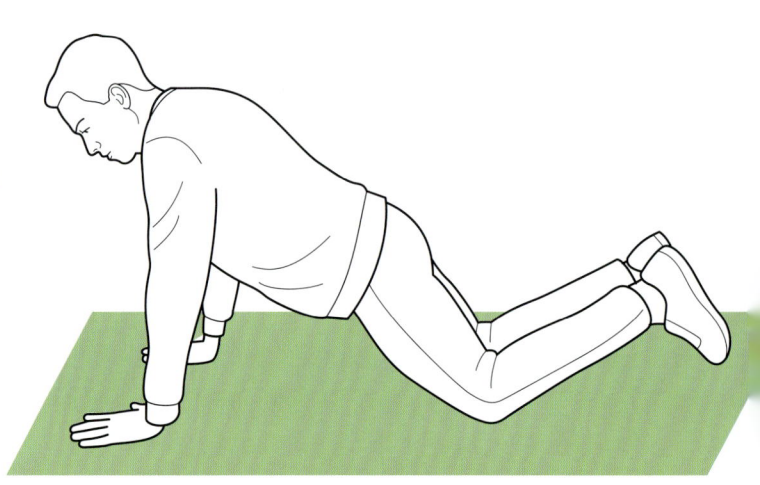

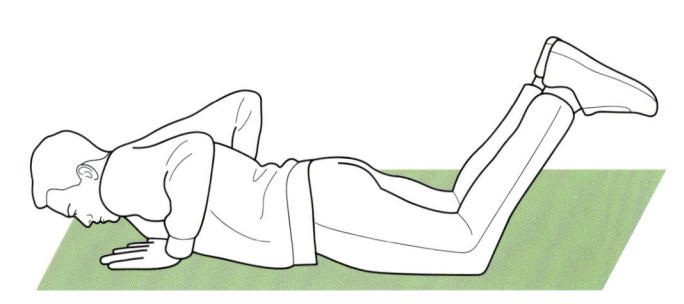

3 KNEELING HAND RELEASE PUSH-UP

Start on all fours with your hands directly under your shoulders, knees bent and feet off the floor. From here, walk your hands forward until the body forms a kneeling push-up position. Engage your tummy muscles and glutes. Lower your chest slowly all the way to the floor, pulling your elbows in towards your side until your chest touches down. From the lower position, briefly lift your hands off the floor. Place them back into push-up position and drive back up to the start position with your core tightened and glutes squeezed. Don't let your hips sag in order to protect your lower back.

Do 6–10 reps keeping excellent form in weeks 1 and 2, increasing to 8–12 reps in weeks 3 and 4. When you can comfortably do 10–12 reps move on to the hand release push-up.

4 HAND RELEASE PUSH-UP

Start in a plank position with your knees off the floor and your hands a bit wider than your shoulders. Control your descent to the floor until your chest makes full contact, maintaining a straight line through your trunk. Briefly lift your hands off the floor. Place them back on the floor and push back up to the starting position.

Do 6–10 reps keeping excellent form in weeks 1 and 2, increasing to 8–12 reps in weeks 3 and 4.

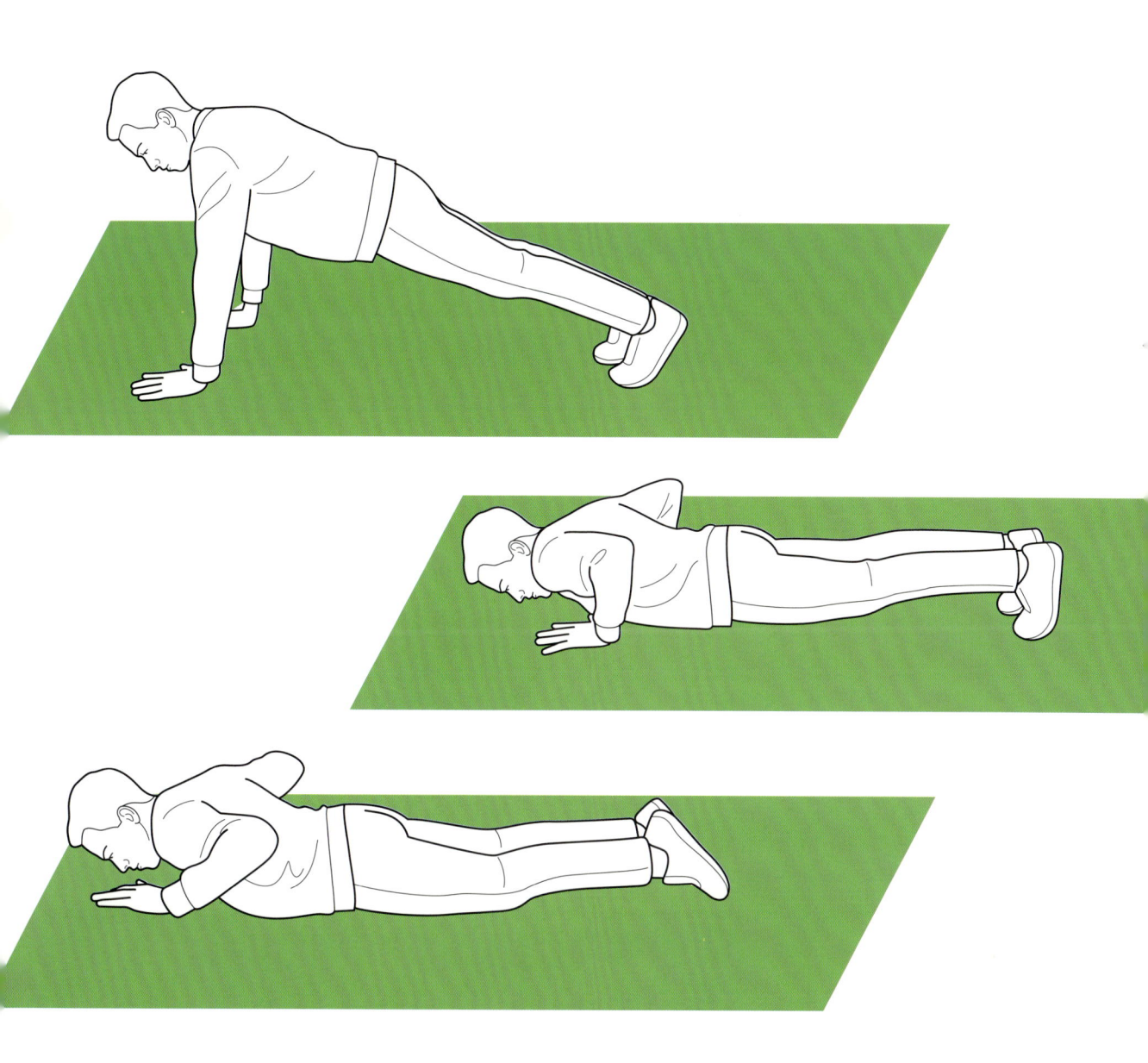

FULL GAS FOREVER

PULL

1 SKYDIVER

Lie on your front with your elbows bent so that your arms are at a 90-degree angle to your trunk. Lift your arms and chest slightly off the floor, focusing on squeezing your shoulder blades together and engaging your glutes and spinal muscles. Hold for 10 seconds before lowering down to the start position.

Do 2–3 reps of 10 seconds in week 1, increasing to 2 x 15 seconds in weeks 2 and 3, and aiming for a 30-second hold in week 4.

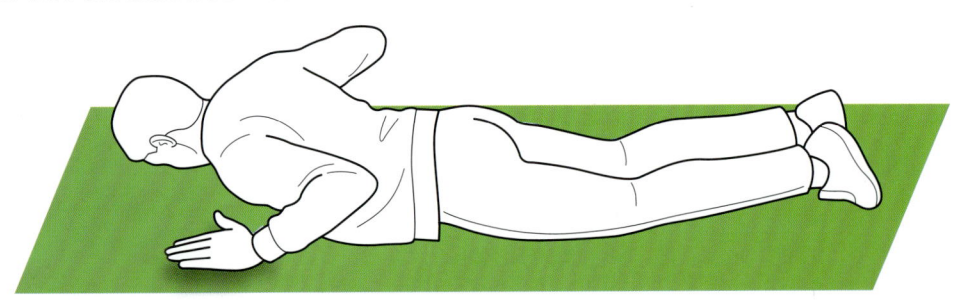

2 FLOOR SWIMMER

Get into the skydiver position, but this time you're going to move your arms. Draw the elbows in towards your sides, maintaining that squeeze between the shoulder blades and glutes. From this position, reach your hands overhead as far as feels comfortable, holding that tension through the shoulder blades, spine and glutes.

Do 6–8 reps in week 1, 8–10 reps in weeks 2 and 3, and 10–12 reps in week 4.

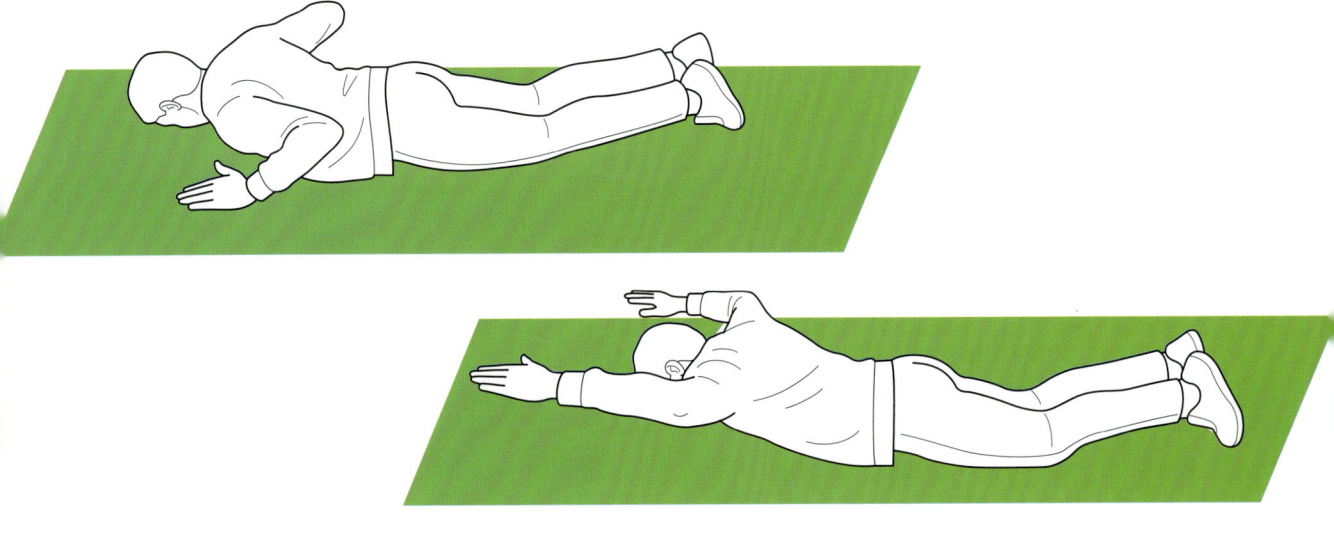

STRENGTH TRAINING

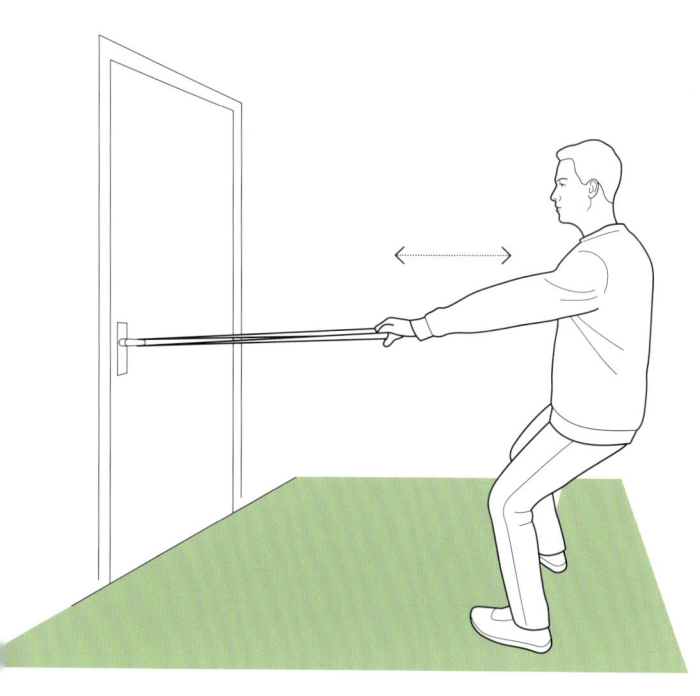

3 STANDING SINGLE ARM ROW VIA A DOOR FRAME

Use a resistance cable that hooks over a door handle. Attach one end around the door handle, ensuring the door is fully closed. Step back to add some tension to the cable, standing with your feet shoulder-width apart and with a small bend in the knees. From here, one arm performs the rowing action while you keep your hips and chest facing forward. Imagine your shoulder blade is being drawn back and down into your opposite trouser pocket. Try not to shrug your shoulder.

Do 8–10 reps per side (starting on your non-dominant side) in weeks 1 and 2, working up to 10–12 reps per side in weeks 3 and 4.

ANTERIOR CHAIN (front of body)

1 BODYWEIGHT SQUAT

Start standing with your feet slightly wider than shoulder-width apart and rotated out between 5 and 10 degrees. Squat as if sitting back into a chair, maintaining control as you lower down. Your chest should stay tall, as if showing off a logo to someone in front of you, until you reach your comfortable squat depth. From the lowest position, think about standing up fast while maintaining control, to get the most out of the exercise. Your feet should remain flat on the floor the whole time.

Do 8–10 reps in weeks 1 and 2, and 10–12 reps in weeks 3 and 4.

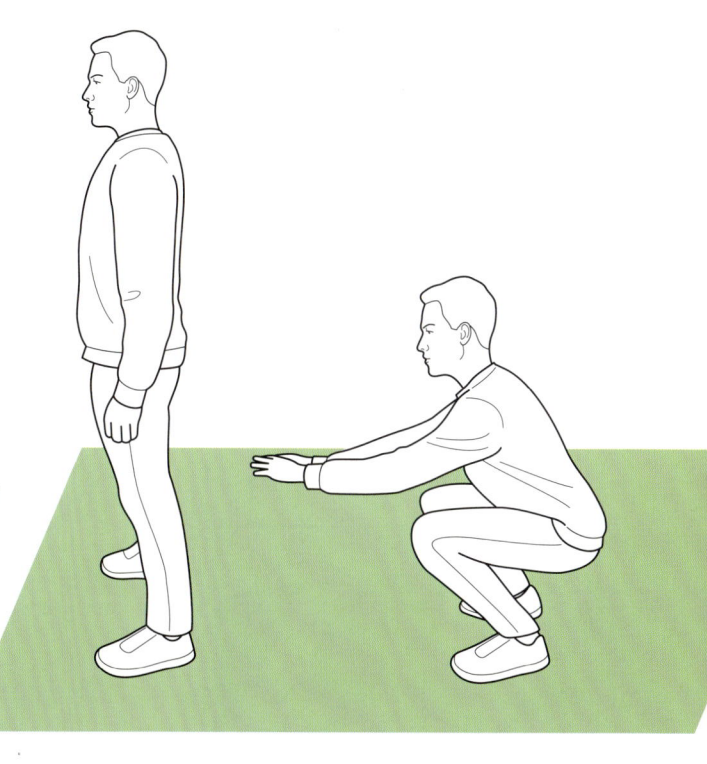

FULL GAS FOREVER

2 STATIC SPLIT SQUAT

Start standing with your feet under your hips. Step one foot back behind you as if taking a moderate stride backwards. Remain on the ball of your foot for this leg, with your heel pointing straight up towards the sky without any rotation out or in. Place your hands on your hips and, maintaining control, lower your back knee down towards the floor until it lightly touches the surface, keeping your front foot flat and your chest tall. From here, drive up through your front leg until you reach the starting position. Ensure you are stable and balanced throughout the movement. It's vital your hips face forwards during this movement.

Aim for 6–8 reps per side in weeks 1 and 2, increasing to 10–12 reps per side in weeks 3 and 4.

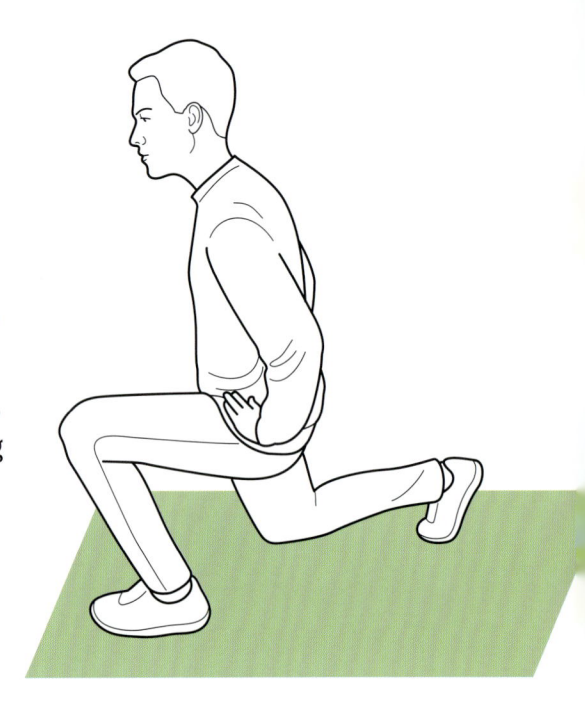

3 REVERSE LUNGE

Start standing with your feet under your hips. Step one foot back behind you as if taking a moderate stride backwards and lower your knee to the floor (similar to the split squat). At the bottom of the movement, instead of just coming up, step your back foot all the way in to return to the start position. This adds a dynamic component to the exercise, further challenging stability and control. Keep your chest tall, with your hips facing forwards, and ensure your front foot remains flat on the floor. Ensure your back knee only brushes the floor, to minimise any risk of impact to your knee.

Aim for 6–8 reps per side in weeks 1 and 2, increasing to 10–12 reps per side in weeks 3 and 4.

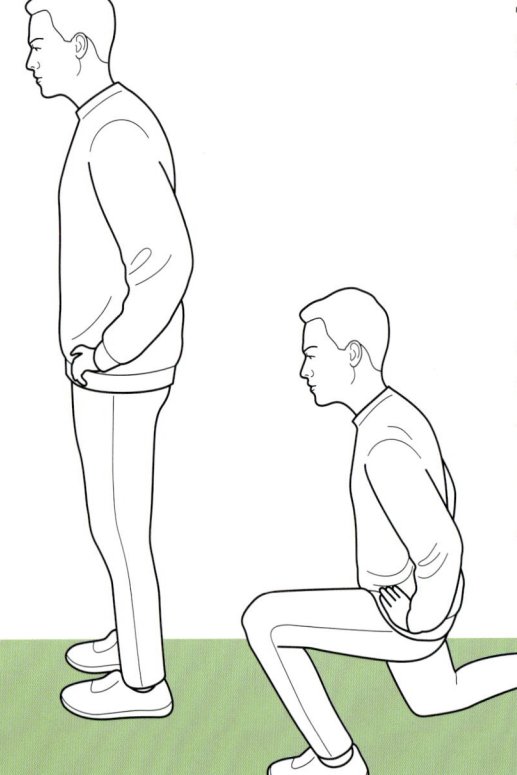

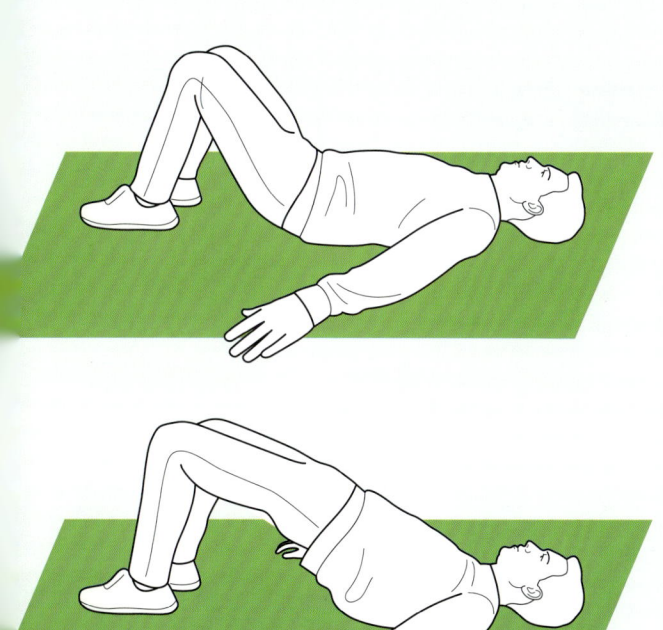

STRENGTH TRAINING

POSTERIOR CHAIN (back of body)

GLUTE BRIDGE

Lie on your back with your legs bent and your feet flat on the floor, hip-width apart, with your arms by your sides. Slowly raise your hips until your torso makes a straight line from your shoulders to your knees. At the top position, squeeze your glutes together while tensing your tummy tightly. Lower your hips back to the floor.

Do 8–10 reps in weeks 1 and 2, and 10–12 reps in weeks 3 and 4.

HAMSTRING BRIDGE

Lie on your back close to a chair or sofa and place your heels on the chair so that your legs form a 90-degree angle. Flex your feet so your toes point upwards. Drive down through your heels to lift your hips up off the chair, feeling your hamstrings engaging early on, with your glutes activating later in the movement. Keep working through to the top of the glute bridge position. At the top, squeeze your glutes and tense your tummy tightly. Then gently lower your hips back down to the floor until your hips and lower back make contact.

Do 6–8 reps in week 1, 8–10 reps in weeks 2 and 3, and 10–12 reps in week 4.

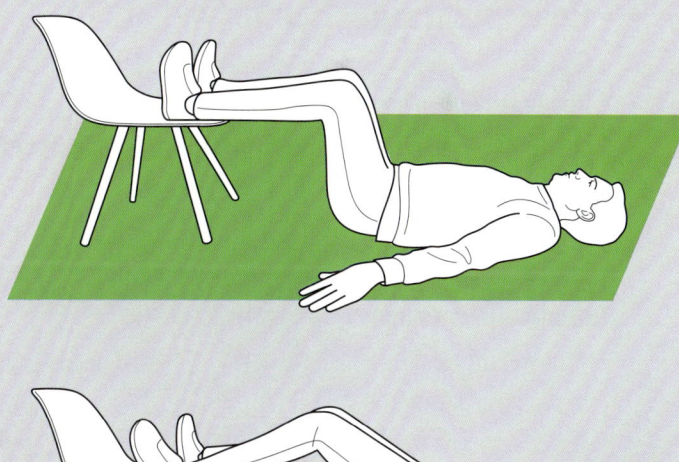

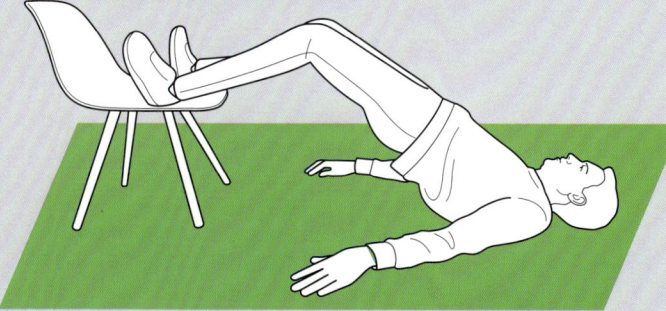

FULL GAS FOREVER

SINGLE LEG HAMSTRING BRIDGE

This exercise is the same as the hamstring bridge, but advancing to a single leg. Initially, it may be a bit tricky to only use one leg for the up and down movement. If this is the case, drive up to the top with both legs, lift one heel off the chair and lower back down with control using a single leg. When you're comfortable with this, this can be advanced to performing the technique with a single leg, both up and down.

Using a single leg places much more load through your hamstrings and back, so target 6 reps per side in week 1, aim for 6–8 reps per side in weeks 2 and 3, and edge up to 8–10 reps per side in week 4.

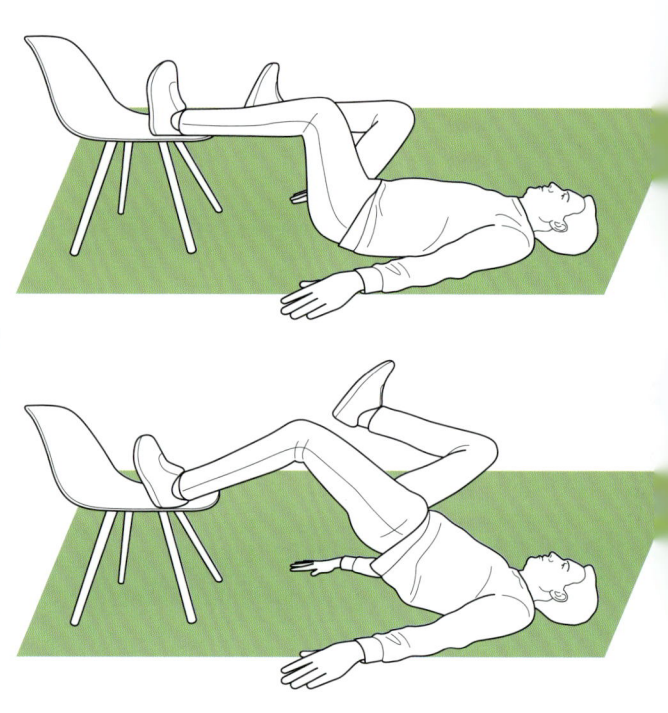

How-to: introduction to weights for cyclists

Ready to pick up some weights? Here are three simple exercises from British Cycling that are ideal for cyclists.

In terms of frequency, twice a week is plenty and when upping the volume of your riding (for example in the summer), bring the frequency of your weight training sessions down to once a week to maintain strength.

How to structure the session

Warm up with light aerobic activity such as running, rowing or spinning the legs on an indoor trainer.

If you are new to weights, just start with 5–6 reps to get used to the movement. Over time, move up to 15–20 reps to challenge yourself. When you are ready to increase the weight, decrease your reps and then repeat the method of increasing the reps over time, and then eventually increasing the weight again.

Cool down at the end of the session by stretching, using a foam roller or repeating the light aerobic activity you did at the start.

STRENGTH TRAINING

A note on reps…

British Cycling advise beginning by doing 4–5 reps to get used to the exercise. Over time, progress the reps to 15–20. Once you are accustomed to doing these higher reps, think about adding more weight, but reducing the number of reps. Then gradually begin adding reps again using your new, heavier weight.

GOBLET SQUAT

This exercise strengthens the muscles around the hips, knees and ankles as well as the postural muscles. Start standing with your feet a little wider than hip-width apart, toes pointing slightly out. Hold a kettlebell or dumbbell close to your chest. Keeping your chest up, squat as if lowering into a chair, driving your knees out. Once you have reached your lowest point while keeping your chest up, pause for a second, then drive up through your feet to return to standing.

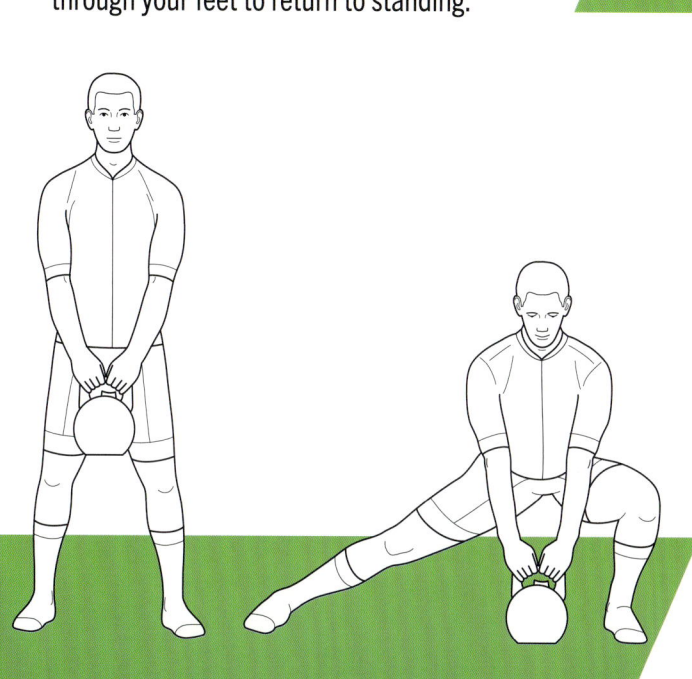

LATERAL SQUAT

This exercise works similar muscles to the goblet squat, but challenges the left and right sides individually (unilaterally). It also improves range of motion. Start standing with your feet much wider than hip-width apart, toes pointing slightly out. Hold a kettlebell or dumbbell down towards the floor with straight arms. Keeping your chest up, step out to the right side, keeping your left leg straight, and bring the weight towards your right foot, with your arms straight. Drive back to the middle.

STIFF LEG DEADLIFT

This exercise works the posterior chain (lower back, glutes and hamstrings). Stand tall with your feet shoulder-width apart and shoulders back. Hold a kettlebell or dumbbell down towards the floor with straight arms. Keep your back straight. Hinge at the hips without moving your knees, and keep pushing your hips back until you feel pressure on your heels and down the back of your hamstrings. Keep your neck in line with your back. Hold for a second, then come back up to standing.

Cycling and weights: the rules

OK, they're not 'rules' as such, but here are some nuggets about how and when to integrate resistance training into your routine. This is more relevant when you start lifting weights as opposed to just doing the bodyweight exercises, because using weights will have more of an impact on your precious legs.

1. Avoid using weights the day before a full-on cycling session such as hill intervals/sprint intervals or racing, because lower-body fatigue from resistance training can persist for up to 24 hours.
2. Preserve your rest days. How many rest days a week you have is highly dependent on your training schedule, but common sense says not to hammer the weight training on every rest day. Have at least one day when your legs can truly rest. If you have a heavy cycle training schedule and are wondering, 'When the hell do I fit it in?', then the next bit of advice might provide a solution.
3. You can cycle and weight train on the same day. But do the bike session first, followed by your weight training session later in the day. How much later depends on the duration and intensity (and hence fatigue) of the bike session. If it was a biggie, push the weight session a bit later and lower the intensity of your weight session.
4. Avoid training the same muscle group on consecutive days. If you do two days of lower body-focused weight training then your legs will be toast before you even start riding.

'The gym just wasn't done'

Back in the day, the gym just wasn't done by endurance cyclists. We stretched and occasionally did a few planks, but strength training was never really discussed. It's always divided opinion and still does today.

The track sprinters do 80 per cent of their training in the gym. It's their bread and butter. They are literally weightlifters who ride bikes now and again.

At the opposite end of the spectrum you have the tour climbers. Naturally slow-twitch athletes, they produce very little peak power, even compared to the average cyclist. They are not explosive or strong in the traditional sense. These riders don't want to carry weight by strengthening muscles they don't use; it's just excess baggage.

I think that argument holds up for those top 1 per cent where it's not about being healthy and well-rounded. But for every other pro cyclist it is important to be robust and in general there has been a massive shift in attitudes towards strength training. It is now considered normal for every pro team rider to have a gym assessment to look at the core or leg strength discrepancy.

A lot of these riders go to the gym pre-season to do the classic exercises for cyclists: leg presses and squats, although it's tricky for them to drop a big strength phase in there because cycling is now a year-round sport thanks to events like the Tour Down Under.

Of course, there's always the odd rider who goes off and does great things who never touches a weight, but they are the exception these days, rather than the norm.

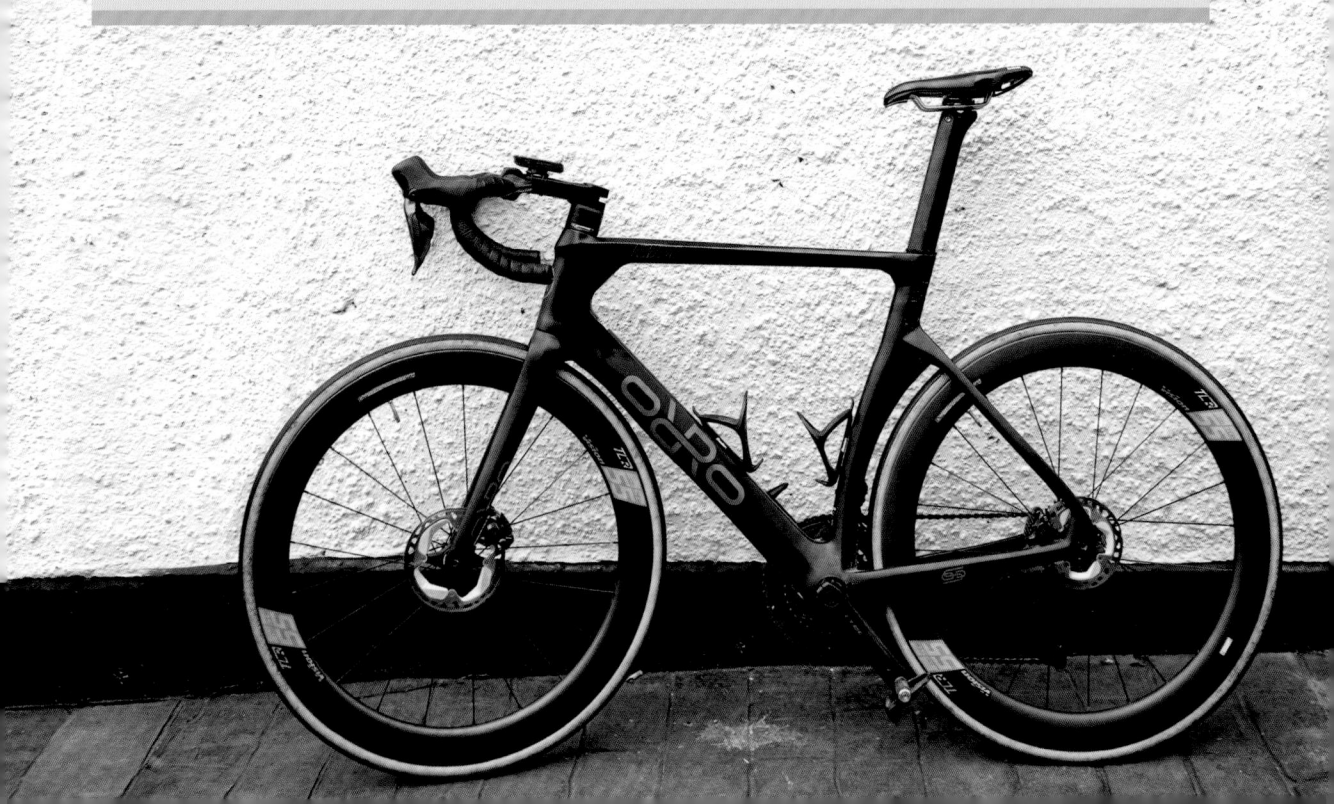

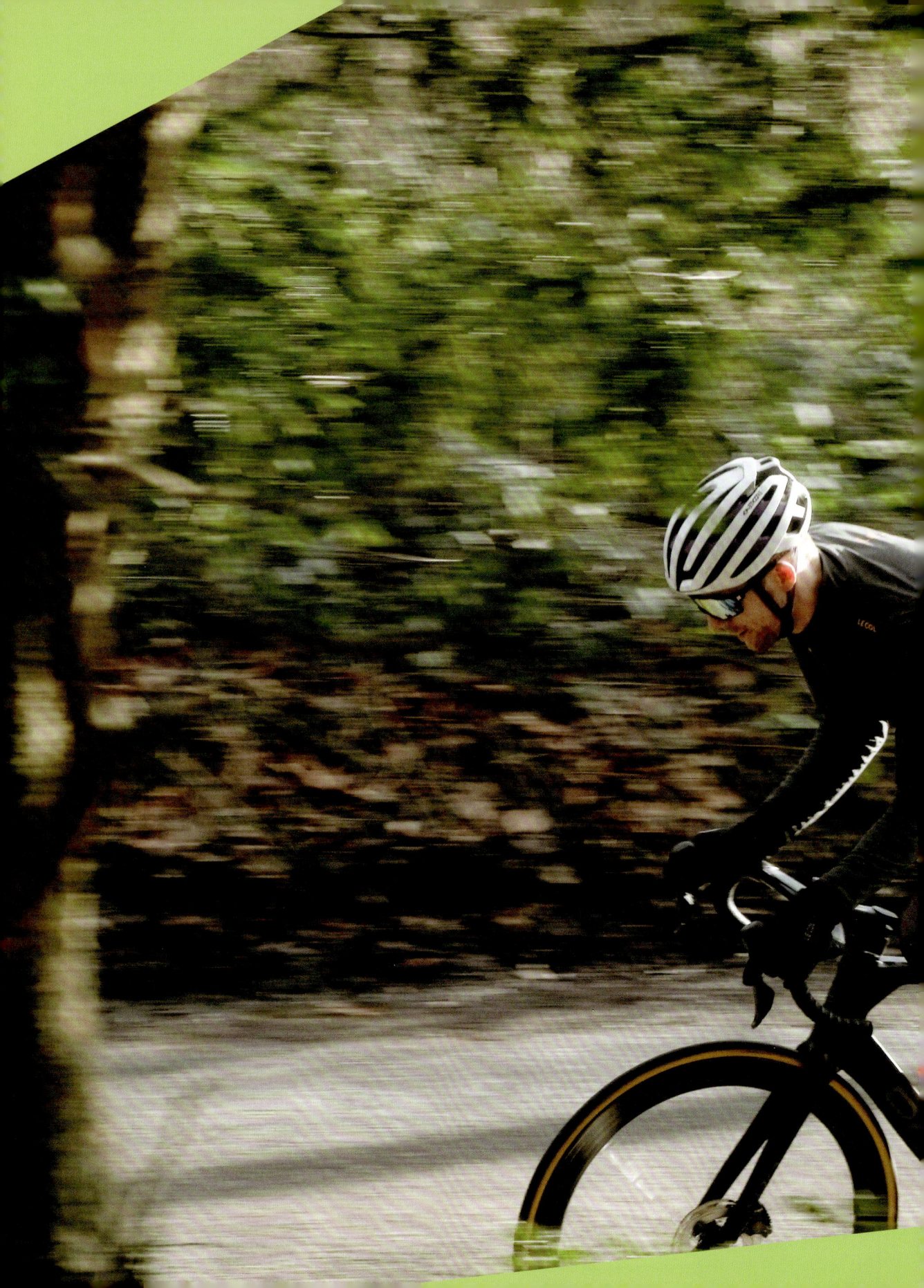

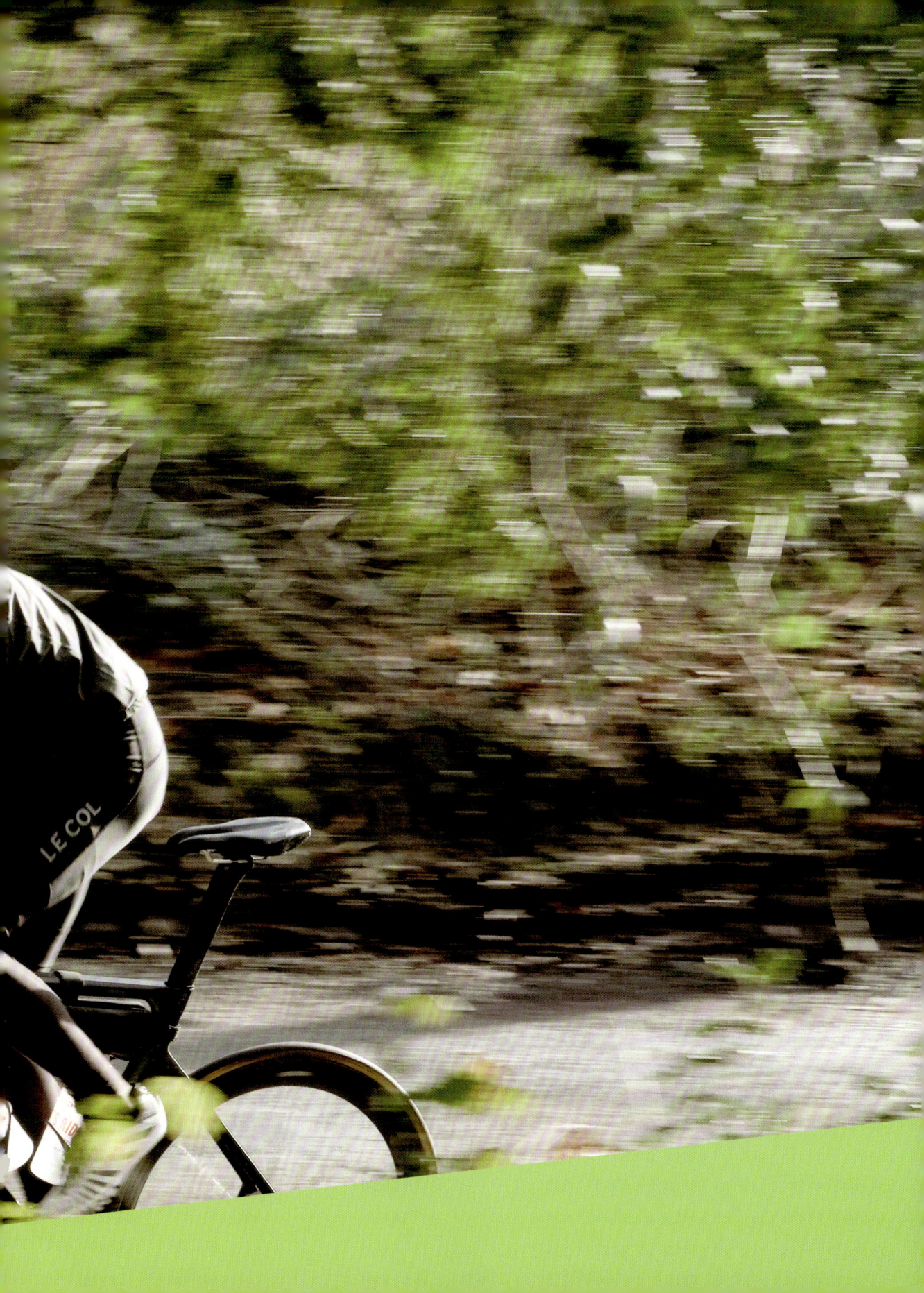

CORE STRENGTH

Lexie Williamson

Cycling is all about legs, legs, legs? Yes and no. Your razor-cut calves and bulging quads are, no doubt, handy for turning the cranks, but the core muscles will channel this leg power and assist with holding an aero position, standing out of the saddle and more. In this chapter we ditch the old-school sit-ups and distil core work down to a handful of bike-specific moves.

The high-performance chassis

Yes, we're not calling it 'the core' any more, but the 'high-performance chassis' (HPC for short); it just sounds sexier. What does it consist of? Well, it's not just that six-pack (it's under there somewhere!), but the entire trunk or torso from your butt all the way up to your shoulders, including the glutes (butt), the traps (neck/shoulder blades), obliques (sides of the torso) and erector spinae (the set of muscles that hold your back up).

A strong HPC will provide the foundation for the work of those strong legs. It's no good having legs of steel if halfway into a big ride your core tires way before your legs, causing your lower back and shoulders to ache and your hips to see-saw in the saddle. Essentially, the core should hold strong and steady, and act as a foundation to enable the legs to power on. Riders with weak cores waste energy that could be channelled into moving them forwards faster.

So, we've established that core strength is essential for cyclists and know it's important for older riders to maintain strength generally, as we lose muscle mass as we age. But 'When am I going to squeeze a core session into my already manic week?', I hear you ask? Fair point and I know you'd much rather be riding your bike. That's why we'll break the techniques down into bite-sized chunks that can be easily consumed.

Some sequences will involve bodyweight only while others use bits and pieces from the gym (kettlebell, dumbbell, stability ball) and so as not to waste your precious riding time, all techniques will be cycling-specific and extend beyond endless reps of

CORE STRENGTH

Lets's stop sucking in that tummy for the group ride photo and put some effort into core work.

sit-ups to encompass the range of muscles required for a bullet-proof core. So, let's stop sucking in that tummy for the group ride photo and put some effort into core work. You only have to do two or three sessions a week before you'll notice a difference.

What constitutes the core?
The core/trunk/torso is a bit like one of those Victorian corsets. It starts at the buttocks (glutes) and back (erector spinae), wrapping around the sides of the waist (internal and external obliques), covering the tummy (transversus abdominis and rectus abdominis), and extends all the way up to the shoulder blades (trapezius). None of these muscles work in isolation so the ideal exercises for cyclists encourage the interaction of these multiple muscle groups.

Four reasons to kick-start that core

1. A strong core minimises energy-wasting rocking in the saddle.
2. A strong core helps you to resist that slump into the saddle on long rides.
3. A strong core helps prevent overuse injuries (knees etc.).
4. A strong core aids pedalling out of the saddle.

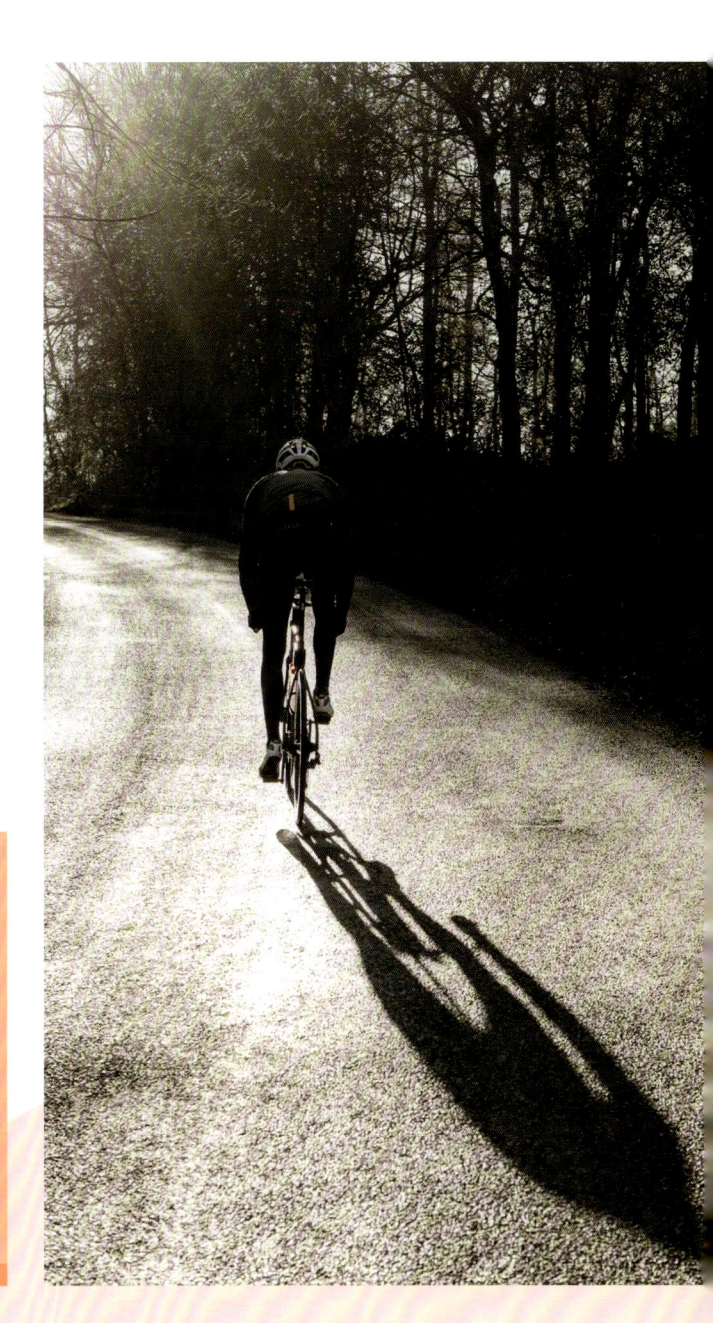

FULL GAS FOREVER

Four do-anywhere core exercises

The beauty of these is that they can be done anywhere! So, no excuses. In an ideal world, you'd perform them three times per week.

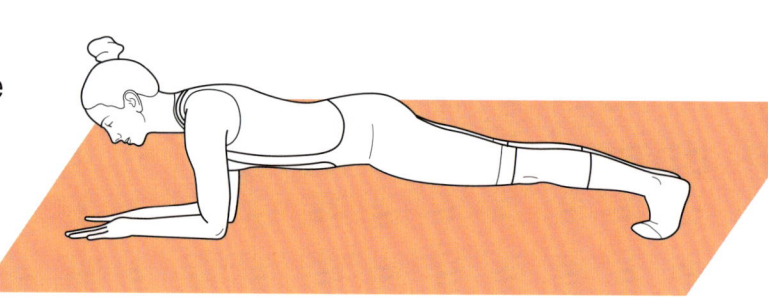

1) FOREARM PLANK

You can't beat plank as a pure core (and more) strength exercise. It's so simple and easy to do, and is also great for building muscular endurance in the drops in an aero position. Try to do a plank at least three times a week and hold for 60 seconds, but you could start with 30 seconds and build up if you need to. To do one, lie on your stomach on the floor with your palms on the floor in front of your shoulders, your elbows tucked in to your sides and the underside of your forearms flat on the floor. Tuck your toes under and push up from your forearms, keeping them flat on the floor. Your body should be raised off the floor in a straight line. Keep your abs engaged and your back straight to avoid the classic sag in the middle of the body.

Hold for 30 seconds, then 1 minute, and build up to 2 minutes over time.

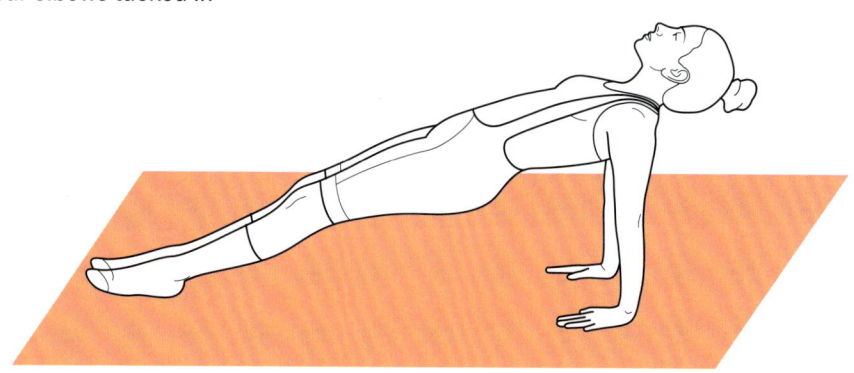

2) REVERSE TABLETOP

This exercise will strengthen your gluteus maximus (the largest butt muscle) and improve stability in the pelvic area, allowing you to achieve a more powerful pedal stroke. Sit on your bottom with your legs bent and your feet flat on the floor, hip-distance apart. Place your hands behind you with your fingers pointing towards your feet. Raise your hips up until they're level with your shoulders and knees, to form a tabletop shape, and squeeze your glutes. Lower back down.

Repeat four more times.

3) SIDE PLANK ROTATION

This is a great one for creating pelvic stability and training the back muscles and oblique (side of tummy) muscles. Come on to your side with your body in a straight line. Position the bottom arm so that you are resting on your forearm, which should be at 90 degrees to your body. Stack your legs so they are one on top of the other, then push up on to the side of the bottom foot, lifting your entire side body off the floor so you are resting on your bottom foot and forearm. Raise your top arm up to the ceiling, then twist towards your forearm on the floor and reach your top hand under your waist. Hold for a couple of seconds, then twist back to the starting position.

Repeat three more times, then turn around to work the other side.

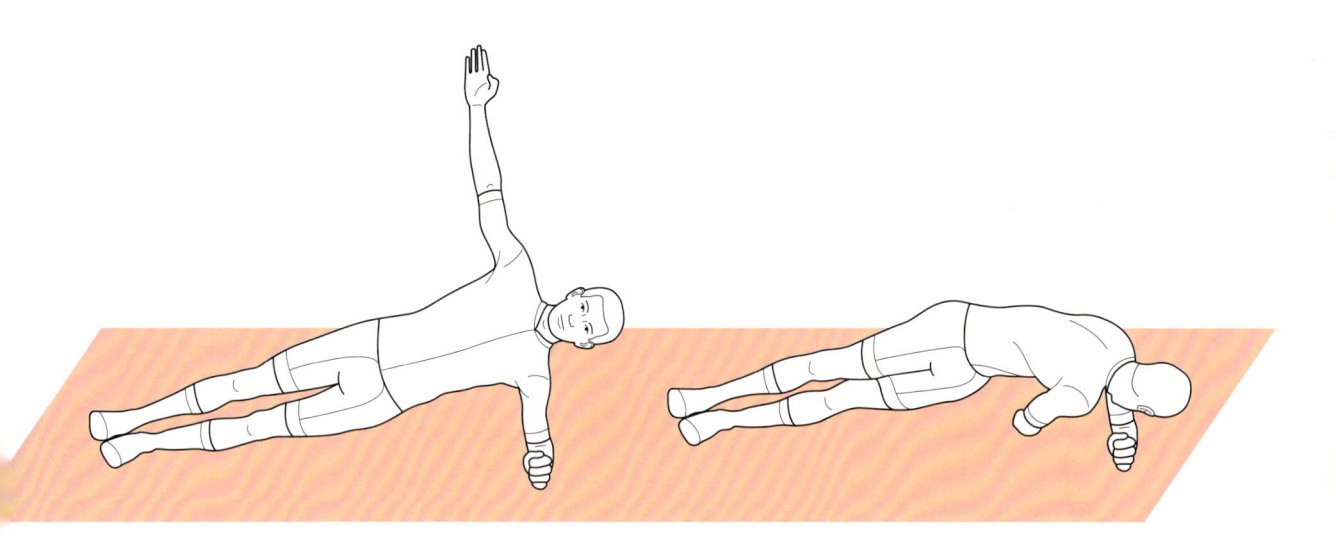

4) PARACHUTE LIFTS

Here's an easy way to fire up the hamstring, glute and lower back muscles (part of the 'posterior chain' in physio lingo). Simply lie on your front with your arms bent into a W shape, palms facing downwards. Keeping your tummy pressed into the floor, lift your arms, legs, chest and neck up into the air. Hold for a second, then lower down.

Repeat four more times.

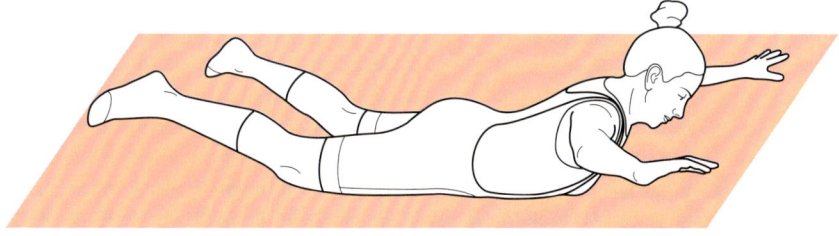

FULL GAS FOREVER

Three easing-in options

Are you looking for a gentler way to work the trunk? Here are some variations on the classic core exercises that either keep the weight off your wrists or place minimal strain on your lower back while getting you working on core stability.

ROLLING BRIDGES

Lie on your back with your legs bent and your feet flat on the floor. Press your lower back into the floor, then lift your backside off the floor and roll your spine off the floor vertebra by vertebra until your hips are high. Slowly lower the spine back down again. Visualise each vertebra as a link in a bicycle chain and try to place each one down one by one.

Repeat four times.

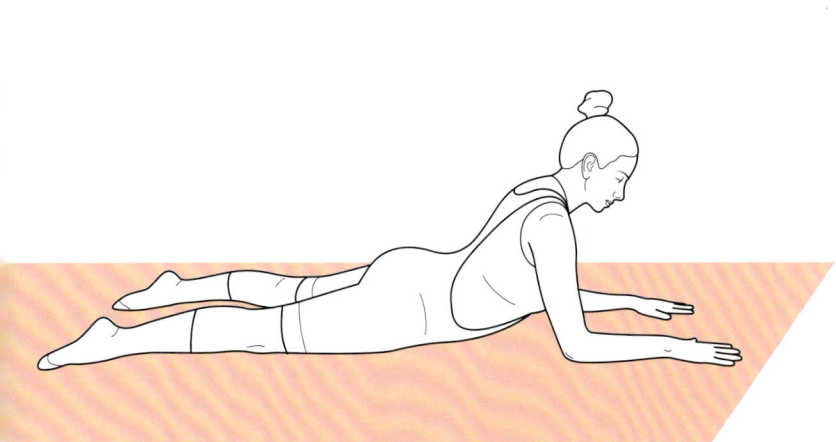

2) SPHINX CRUNCHES

Lie flat on your belly on the floor with your elbows directly underneath your shoulders and your forearms flat on the floor in front of you. Now lift your belly, hips and knees off the floor, and round or flex your spine. Hold for a second, then return to the start position.

Repeat five times.

CORE STRENGTH

3) BENT-LEG WINDSCREEN WIPERS

Lie on your back with your legs bent into a 90-degree position and your arms out to the sides on the floor, level with your shoulders. Lower your knees across to the right and hover them above the floor (or higher if necessary) for a few seconds.

Repeat on the left side and continue swaying the legs slowly from side to side four more times.

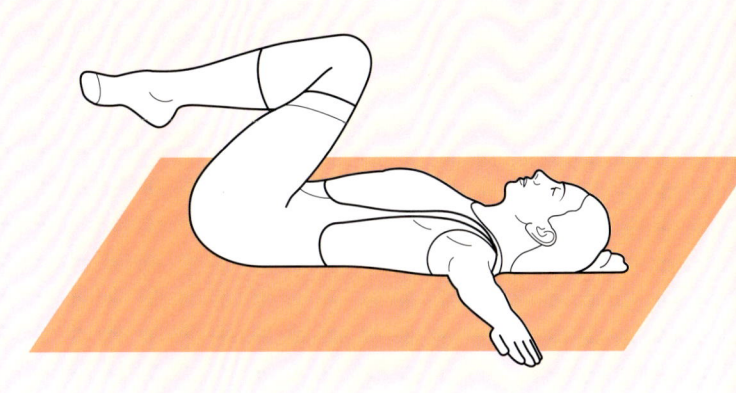

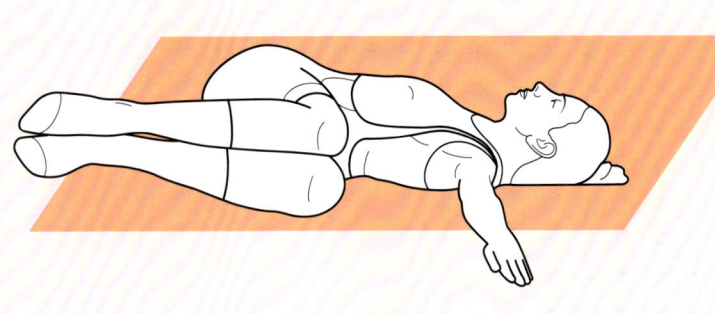

4) LATERAL LEG LIFTS

Lie on your side with your body straight. Stack your legs so they are one on top of the other. Raise both legs off the floor and hold for a second, then lower.

Repeat five more times. An even gentler version of this would be to raise just the top leg.

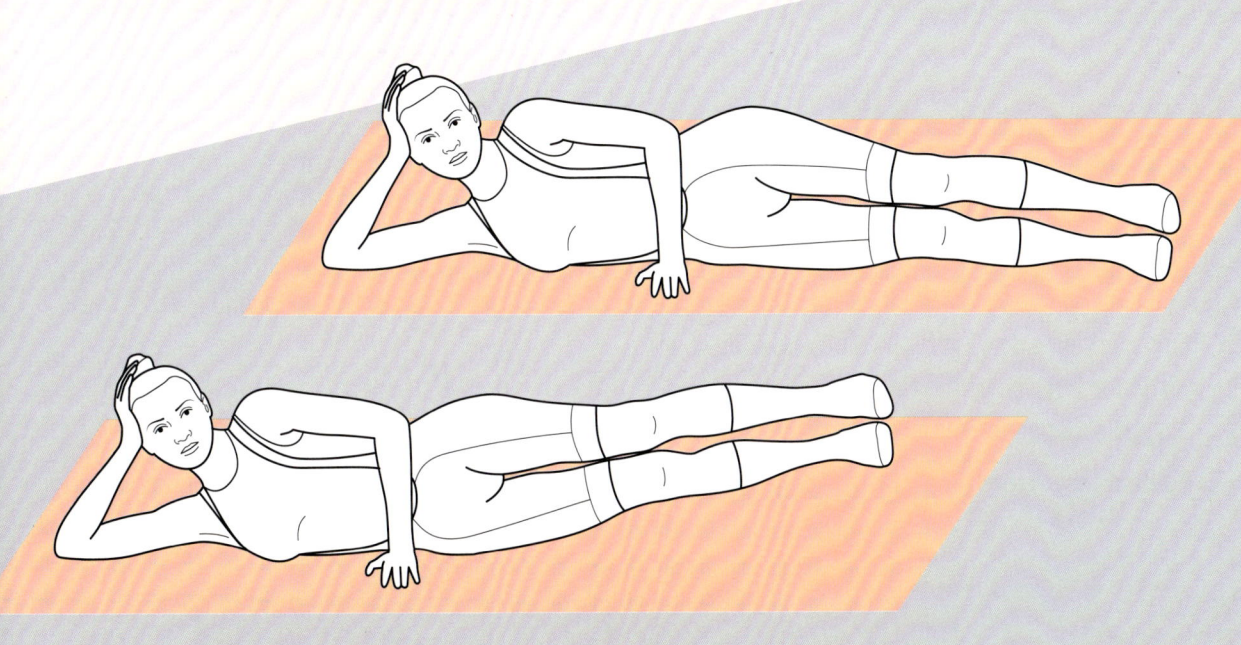

FULL GAS FOREVER

Three gym-based core exercises

Built up your base with bodyweight core exercises? Once you are comfortable with doing those you can move on to these three exercises to do in the gym.

1) STABILITY BALL MOUNTAIN CLIMBER

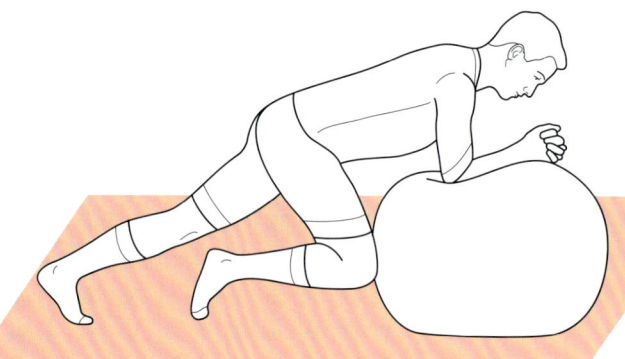

Stability balls create wobbliness and this instability makes the core work even harder. Perform a forearm plank (*see* p. 44) on the ball, ensuring your body is nice and straight. Tap one knee to the ball, then the other.

Continue alternating legs for 1 minute.

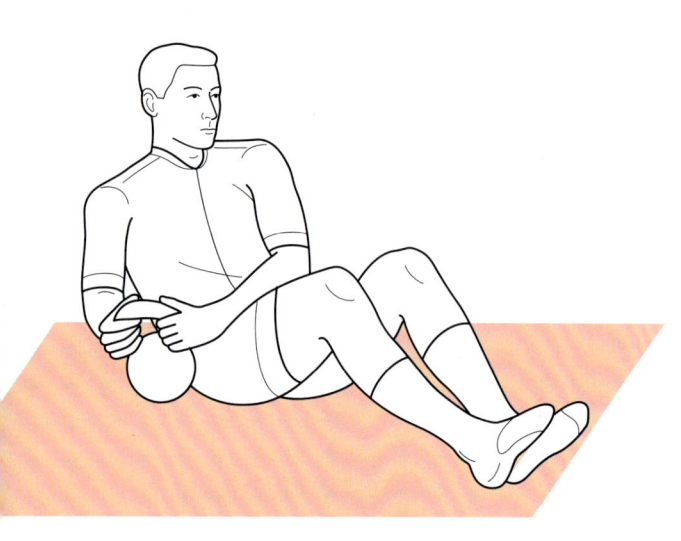

2) RUSSIAN TWIST

Sit on the floor with your legs bent and your heels on the floor. Hold a kettlebell or dumbbell (start with a 4kg/8lb one if you're new to using weights) in front of your chest. Lean back to a 45-degree angle. Rotate your torso to the right and touch the kettlebell or dumbbell to the floor. Return to the centre and rotate to the left side.

Repeat three more times on each side.

3) DUMBBELL SIDE BEND

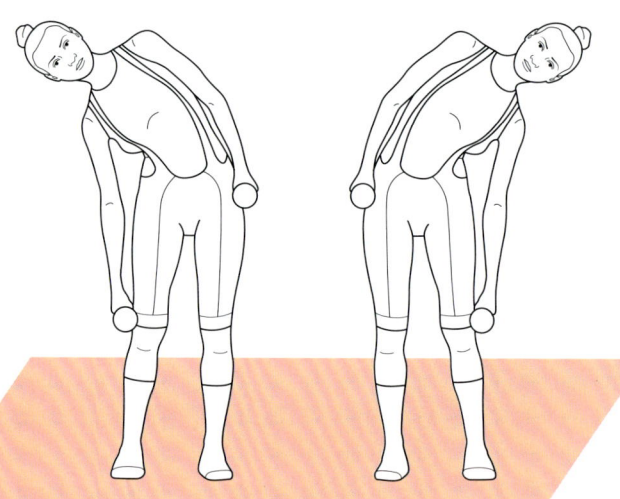

Stand up straight with your feet hip-width apart. Hold a dumbbell in each hand and position your arms by your sides. Tilt to the right and slide your right dumbbell down the side of your leg and back up again. Repeat on the left side.

Repeat three more times on each side.

CORE STRENGTH

Getting aero

If you struggle to get aero on the road bike, this might be down to spinal stiffness. Or do you need help comfortably holding the position on your TT? If either of these is you, try this combination of flexibility and core strength exercises. These techniques activate and build your core, improve flexibility in the thoracic (mid) spine and stretch the hamstrings as they work in a lengthened position on the TT.

1) BIRD DOG

Lie on your back 'dead bug' style with your arms reaching straight up to the ceiling and legs bent to a 90-degree angle. Press your lower back to the floor. Extend the opposite arm and leg by straightening your right leg and reaching your left arm straight overhead, hovering both above the floor. Bring your limbs back to your body and switch to the other side.

Continue for 20 seconds.

2) FOREARM PLANK INTO PLANK

Get into forearm plank position (*see* p.44) and simply move up and down, from your forearms up to full plank on your hands and back down, aiming to minimise rotation of your torso and keeping your core engaged. Make the movement smooth and steady.

Continue for 20 seconds.

If you struggle to get aero on the road bike, this might be down to spinal stiffness.

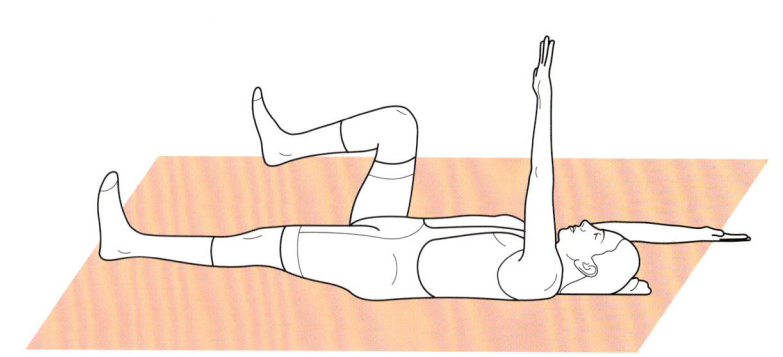

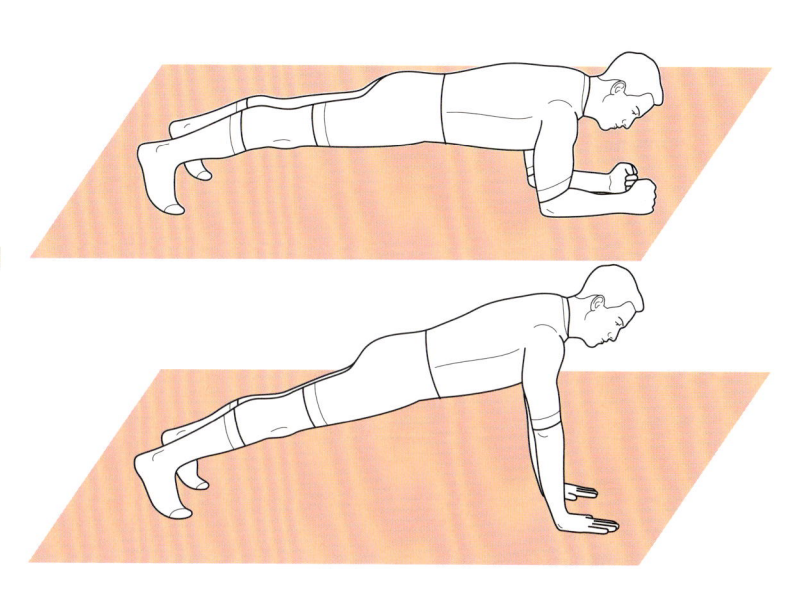

FULL GAS FOREVER

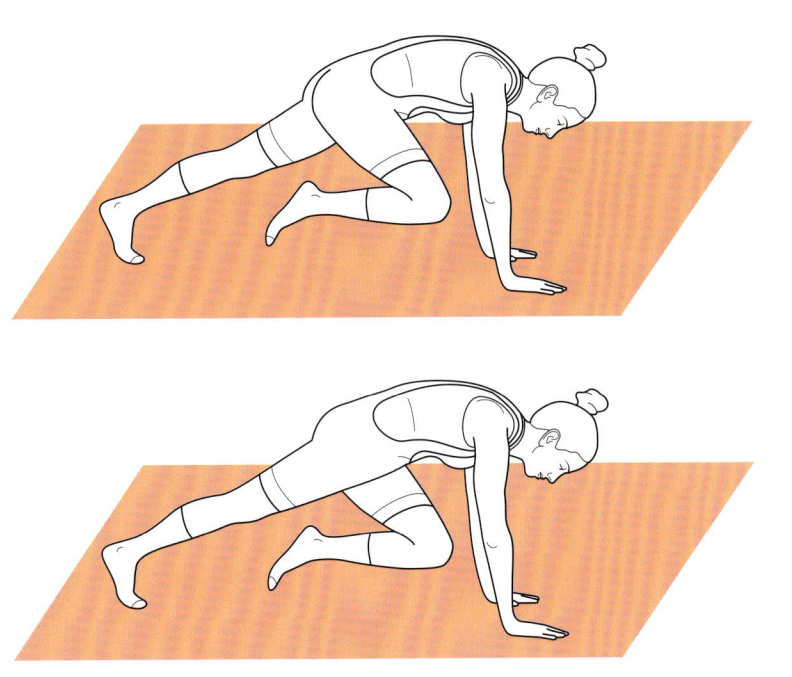

3) STATIC MOUNTAIN CLIMBERS

Get into full plank position (see p.49). Draw your right leg in to the middle of your chest and pause for a few seconds. Return the leg to the start position, then repeat with the left leg. Keep your back still and stable.

Continue for 20 seconds.

4) SEATED CAT STRETCH

Sit with your legs bent and your feet hip-width apart on the floor. Hold under your knees. As you inhale, sit tall, and as you exhale, lean back until your arms straighten and you really flex your spine. Hold for a few seconds, then return to the start position.

Continue for 20 seconds.

Note: Stiffness in the thoracic region, or mid-back, can be a major barrier to maintaining an aero position. If this is a tight spot for you, try holding the second part of seated cat stretch, bring your feet closer in and wrap your arms around the backs of your thighs. Lean back to deeply stretch the back muscles and take some slow, deep breaths. Try to feel the back muscles expand on the inhale and relax on the exhale.

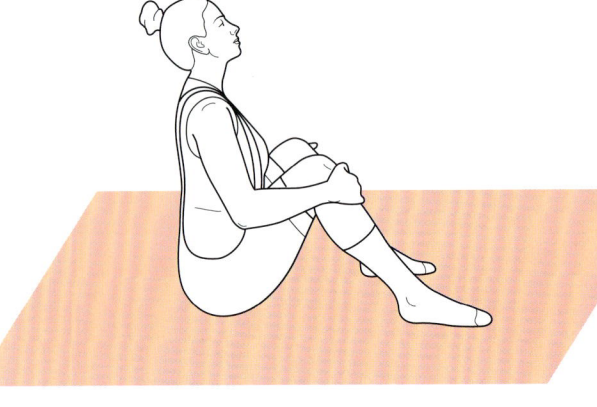

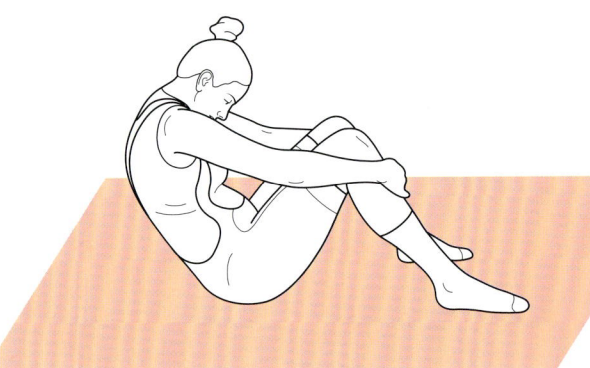

CORE STRENGTH

5) LYING TWIST

Lie flat on your back on the floor. Hug your right leg into your chest. Grab it with your left hand and draw it across your body, until it touches, or nearly touches, the floor to the left of your torso.

Hold for 20 seconds. Repeat on the other side.

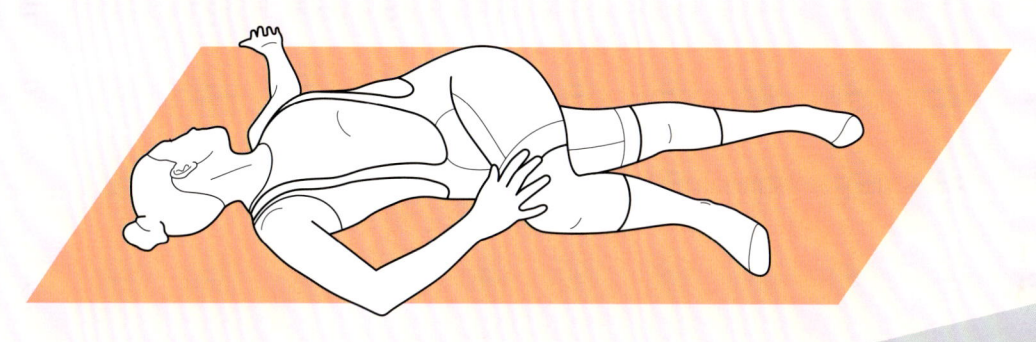

6) STANDING (OR SEATED) FOLD

There are two ways to do this stretch. If you are flexible, sit with your legs stretched out and reach forward. Hold your legs wherever is comfortable (thighs/shins/ankles/grab your feet) and let your spine flex and your head drop down. A gentler version of this is to stand with your legs a little bent and let your upper body fold forwards. Just hang out here, either with your arms dangling or folded.

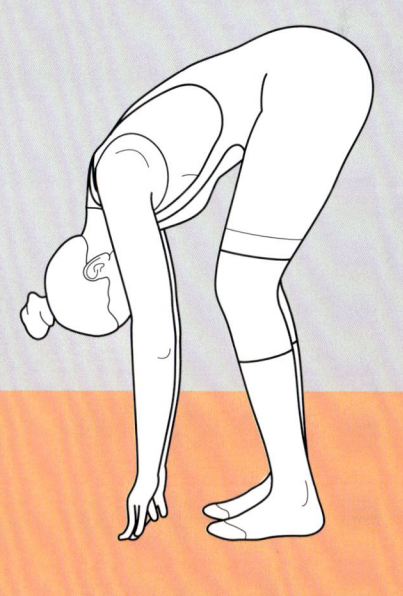

Beat the cycling slump

The flexed cycling stance can take its toll on your posture. Then chuck in the eight hours spent sitting at a desk that many of us have to do in our working lives and a bit of sofa slouching and it all adds up. Posture can also be affected by any of the following:

1. Being sedentary, which leads to muscular atrophy or loss of muscle mass
2. Lack of core strength, as these muscles support your trunk
3. Overuse of certain muscles through a repetitive sport like cycling

The good news is that all the core techniques above will work wonders for bolstering your trunk, which is great for posture, and you can also try these:

1) THORACIC CAT

Start on all fours. Without changing your head position, lift your mid-back up towards the ceiling. Now drop your chest so it sinks towards the floor.

Repeat four more times.

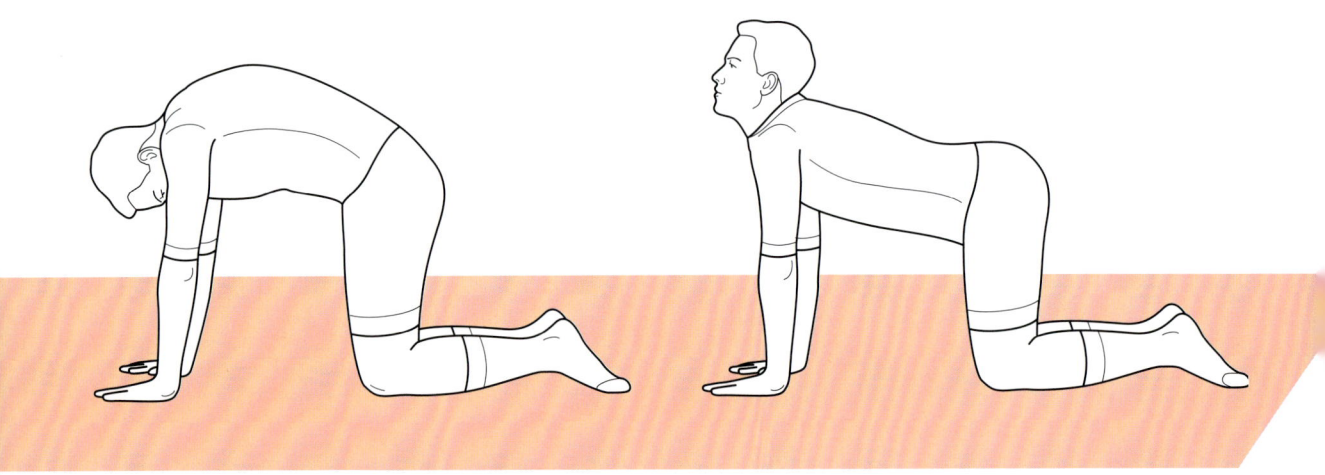

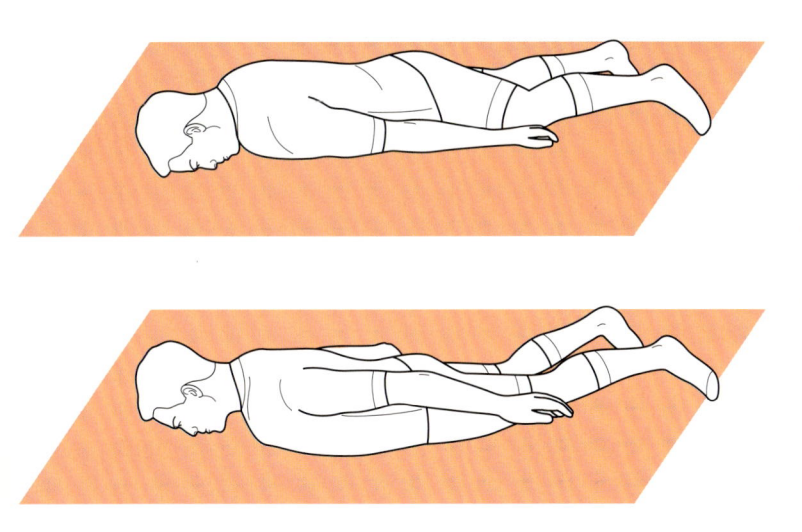

CORE STRENGTH

2) PRONE SNOW ANGELS

Lie face down with your arms by your sides. Lift your arms, legs and as much of your torso as possible off the floor. Sweep your arms out to the sides and overhead in a wide V shape. Now return them to your sides and lower your body back to the floor.

Repeat four more times.

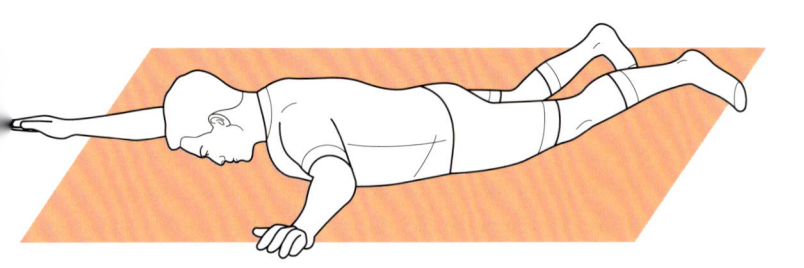

3) STRAP PEC STRETCH

This is a go-to stretch for postural correction. It also just feels amazing post-ride. If you don't have a cotton yoga strap, use a sweatshirt sleeve or rolled-up towel. Hold one end of the strap in each hand and open out your hands, so the strap is pulled taut. Raise the strap overhead until you feel a tugging sensation in your pectoral muscles. Play with bending the arms into a W position or straightening them into a wide V.

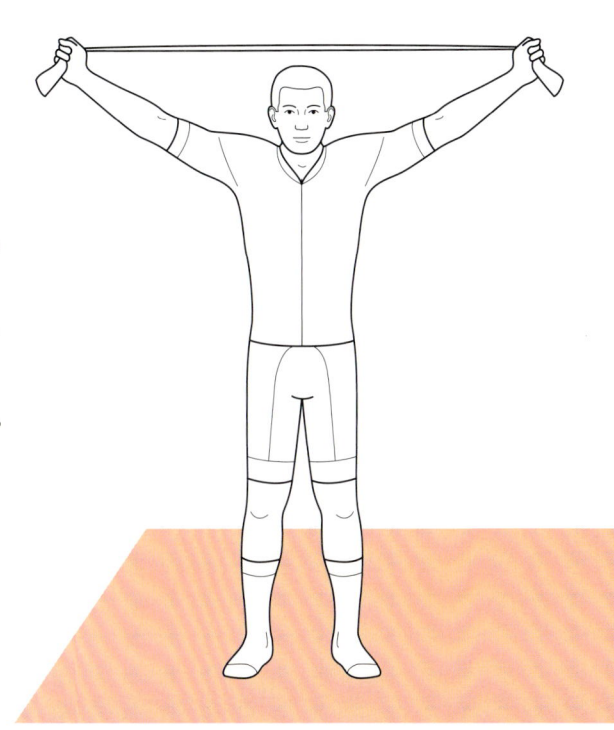

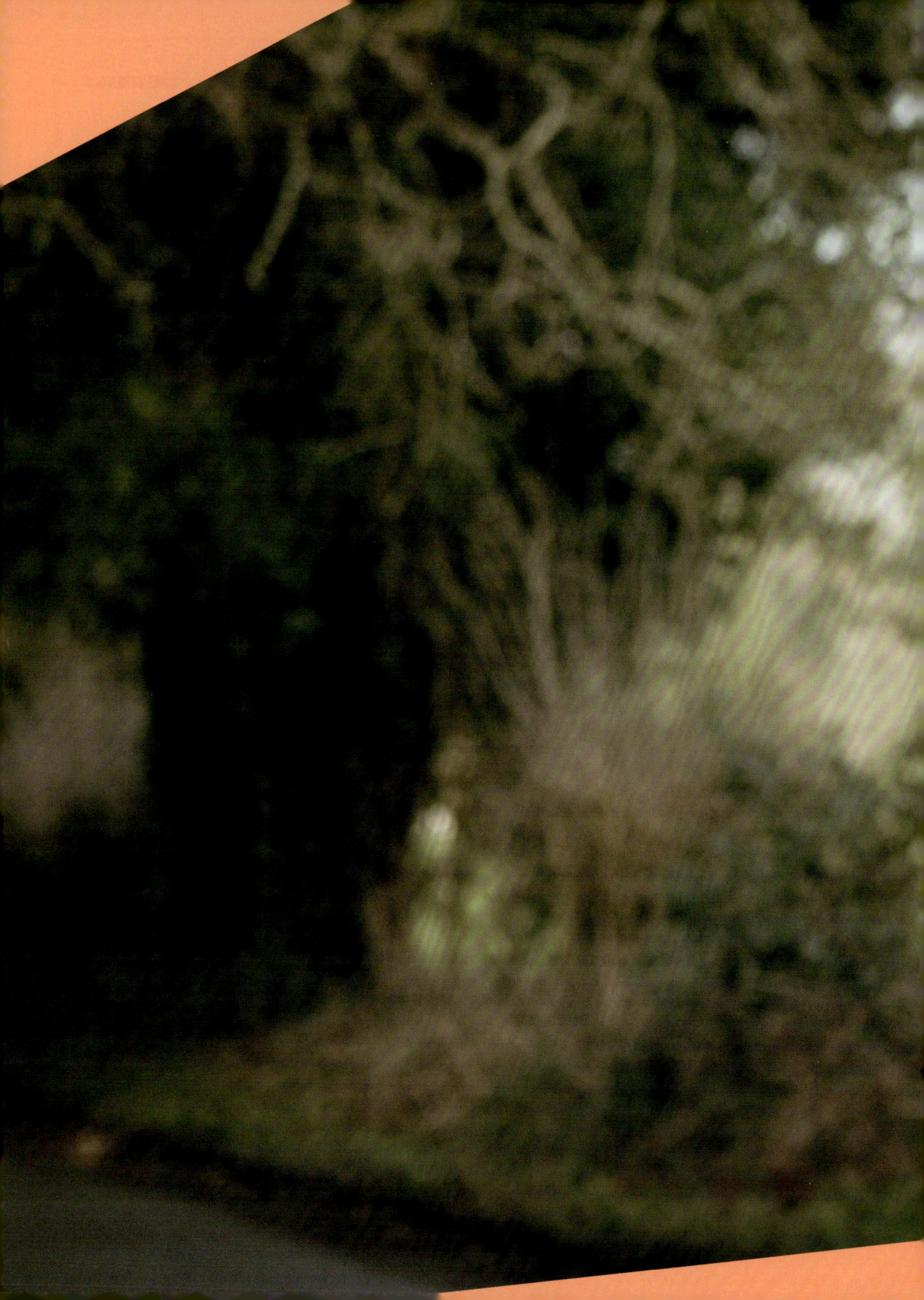

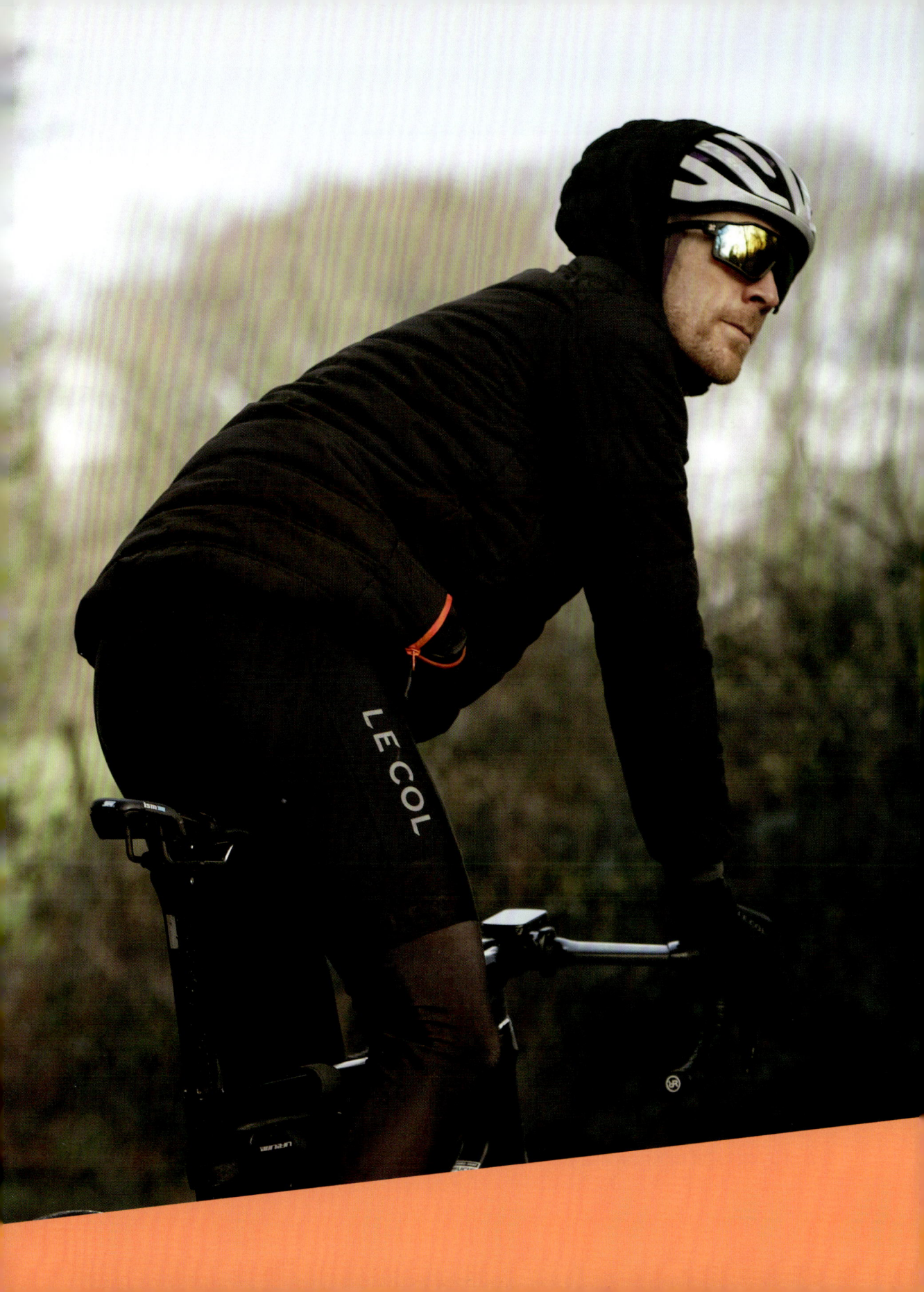

MINIMISING RESISTANCE

Ed Clancy

What's holding you back? Only the air around you. Minimising air resistance as you ride is the key to conserving energy and increasing speed.

Going faster isn't necessarily about spending money. Aerodynamic drag (air resistance) is the biggest external factor affecting a cyclist's performance. On a flat road, by 16km/h (10mph) it is consuming half of your power and by 48km/h (30mph) that reaches around 80 or 90 per cent. Of all this air resistance holding you back, around 75–80 per cent is due to your body. There's no avoiding it; as good a bike as you have, someone's got to ride it. The more you can reduce the drag, the faster you can go. On a 40km (25-mile) time trial, for instance, if you can reduce the aero drag by 10 per cent, it is possible to save 90 seconds or more.

The front of the bike bears the brunt of the air resistance and common sense says the smaller your front profile is, the less resistance you will encounter. A starting point is that if your position looks streamlined, your body made small and compact, then the chances are it is. However, the days of trying to get super low with your arms on the drops have gone. Too much focus on a low front end with very low bars – on either a road or TT set-up – will compromise your hip angle and power. You're often better off having a primary focus on being narrow rather than super low to achieve a small frontal area.

On a road bike, the most aerodynamic position for most people is to have the hands on the hoods, shoulders shrugged narrow, forearms horizontal and your head low. And on TT bikes it's often faster if your hands are raised in front of your chin or lower face. Body positioning is not an exact science – different positions suit different body types – but I've done a lot of work in the wind tunnel and narrower works every time.

As useful as it can be, it doesn't help to become so focused on aerodynamic position that other issues are neglected. Going up hills and mountains is where the real time differences are often gained.

MINIMISING RESISTANCE

I've been on the bikes of Dan Bigham and Charlie Tanfield, both great pursuit riders, and the first thing I noticed was they are comfortable to ride. Even on track bikes ridden for a matter of minutes, comfort and power are key. Getting that balance right is essential. From 2008, when I was in the GB track racing team, aerodynamics kept us ahead of the rest of the world. Since then, other nations and road cycling have caught up. Not just elite riders, but club and recreational cyclists too, are taking their bikes to the wind tunnels and trying out riding positions and clothing. The genie is out of the bottle and there's no going back ….

Bike fit

Seeking professional advice on setting up your bike will give you a good starting point and a window in which to operate. Exactly how you position yourself when you ride is so subjective. However, it is still helpful if someone watches you ride and suggests the optimal height for your bars, crank length or where your saddle should be. If you are buying a new bike, a bike fit is often provided free, so use it as a starting point. That said, if you are buying a new bike, a bike fit is often provided free, so use it as a starting point.

There have been great advances in bike fit apps in recent years, which can provide a really good guide before you buy a bike and are a good starting point when it comes to adjusting an existing bike. Some of the basic apps are free, but even the ones you pay for, which give a more detailed assessment and recommendations, are a fraction of the cost of visiting a professional bike fitter. The process is pretty simple. You input various body measurements and upload short videos of your riding style, and it gives you recommendations of numerous adjustments, including saddle, handlebar and brake hood heights, and positions.

Many riders approaching or well into their middle age will be beginning to feel the effects of ageing and have historical

The smaller your front profile is, the less resistance you will encounter.

Simple saddle-fit 1-0-1

Always get the back end of the bike – saddle and cleat positions – sorted before adjusting the front end.

Wearing your cycling gear, measure your inside leg from your crotch to the top of the sole of your foot. Multiply this by 109 per cent to get your saddle-top to pedal measurement.

Tilt the saddle-nose down 3 or 4 degrees (about 0.5cm/0.2in).

If you have the appropriate frame size you should be able to reach the top of the bar with a slight bend at the elbow and your back at a 45-degree angle.

You should be upright on the tops and comfortable on the drops. If not, change your stem for a longer, shorter, higher or lower one, or insert spacer rings to adjust the stem height.

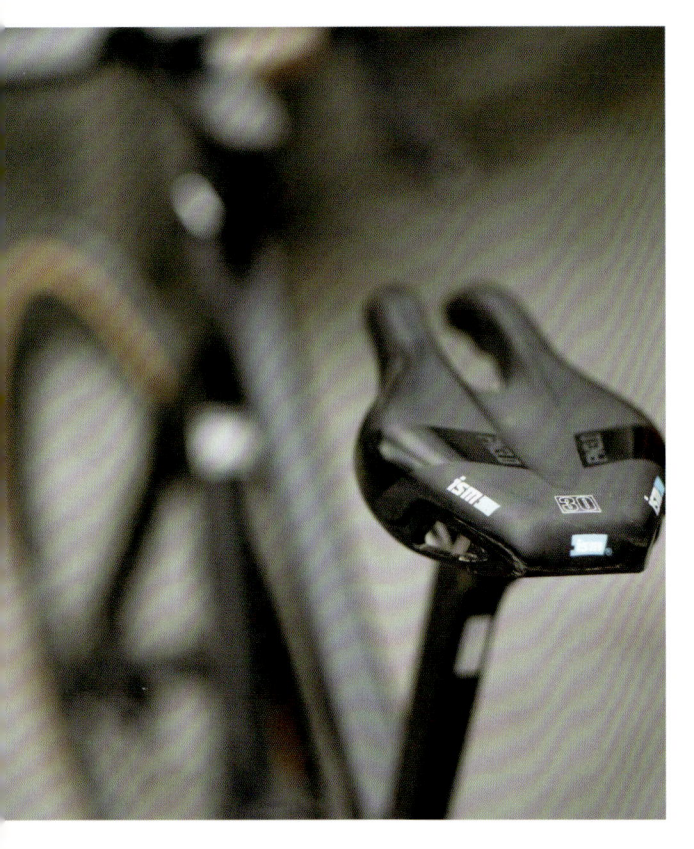

and new strains and injuries to consider. What feels comfortable after 50km (30 miles) can become agony by 80km (50 miles). You might need to make adjustments yourself to suit your riding position and to alleviate any aches or pains, so remember to take some Allen keys with you and keep refining your fit until you know you have it right.

Saddle

It's easy to work out a position for your saddle that will give you a starting position to work from (see 'Simple saddle-fit 1-0-1' above). You will soon know if it's too high, as your hips will start rocking. If it's too low, it will just feel cramped, like you are pushing a wheelbarrow. Spending hours on a bike can make you super-sensitive to the exact height of the saddle. I could sit on a spare bike and instantly know if it was a couple of millimetres out.

That said, the same does not apply to all riders. Respected bike fitter Phil Burt came up with the terms 'micro-adjusters and macro-absorbers', which describe both those riders who can feel the smallest change and those who don't seem to notice or care about relatively big changes. Mark Cavendish is known to regularly change his seat height according to the terrain he's riding, whereas it took Chris Froome three years to discover he had changed his riding position after his major crash in 2019. He ended up changing his saddle height by centimetres.

Handlebars

Those looking for speed should choose the aerodynamic efficiency of narrow bars, as there is very little trade-off with power production and comfort. However, it is all about moderation; I'm not suggesting anyone puts 37cm (14.6in) bars on, otherwise turning capability can become hellish. Experiment first with bars that are 2cm (0.8in) narrower and see how it feels before going to extremes.

The starting point for handlebar height should be about 5cm (2in) lower than the saddle. The bar can then be lowered – maybe 10–15cm (4–6in) lower if you are racing – depending on your preferences. The basic positions of a higher bar for maximum control on a mountain bike and a lower bar for the best aerobic position on a road bike are subject to the demands made by your body shape and riding style. It is easy to adjust, though, according to how comfortable you feel. On a road bike, one simple test is to see how long you spend on the drops. If you are rarely on the hoods and often on the drops then they're probably too high. If it is uncomfortable riding on them for more than a few minutes then maybe they are too low.

Cleats

The feet are the major point of power transfer between you and the bike, so cleat position becomes a major issue. Your foot stability, the muscles used and your ability to sprint can all vary. All feet are different and hours in the saddle can cause all kinds of ankle, knee and hip problems if the cleats are forcing you to pedal in a

Aligning cleats

Set up your cleats so the axle of the pedal is right under the ball of your foot. If necessary, adjust them 15–20mm (0.6–0.8in) backwards from the centre for stability and comfort. Shorter-distance riders and sprinters might position them the same amount forward for sheer power.

Check whether the straight angle is correct for you. Perch on a table or bench with your feet dangling. Observe how much and which way they naturally angle and replicate that angle with the cleat – remember that each foot could angle differently.

Monitor your riding style. If you are not comfortable, your knees are pointing in or out too much, or your heels are too high or low, then adjust the cleats as soon as you can.

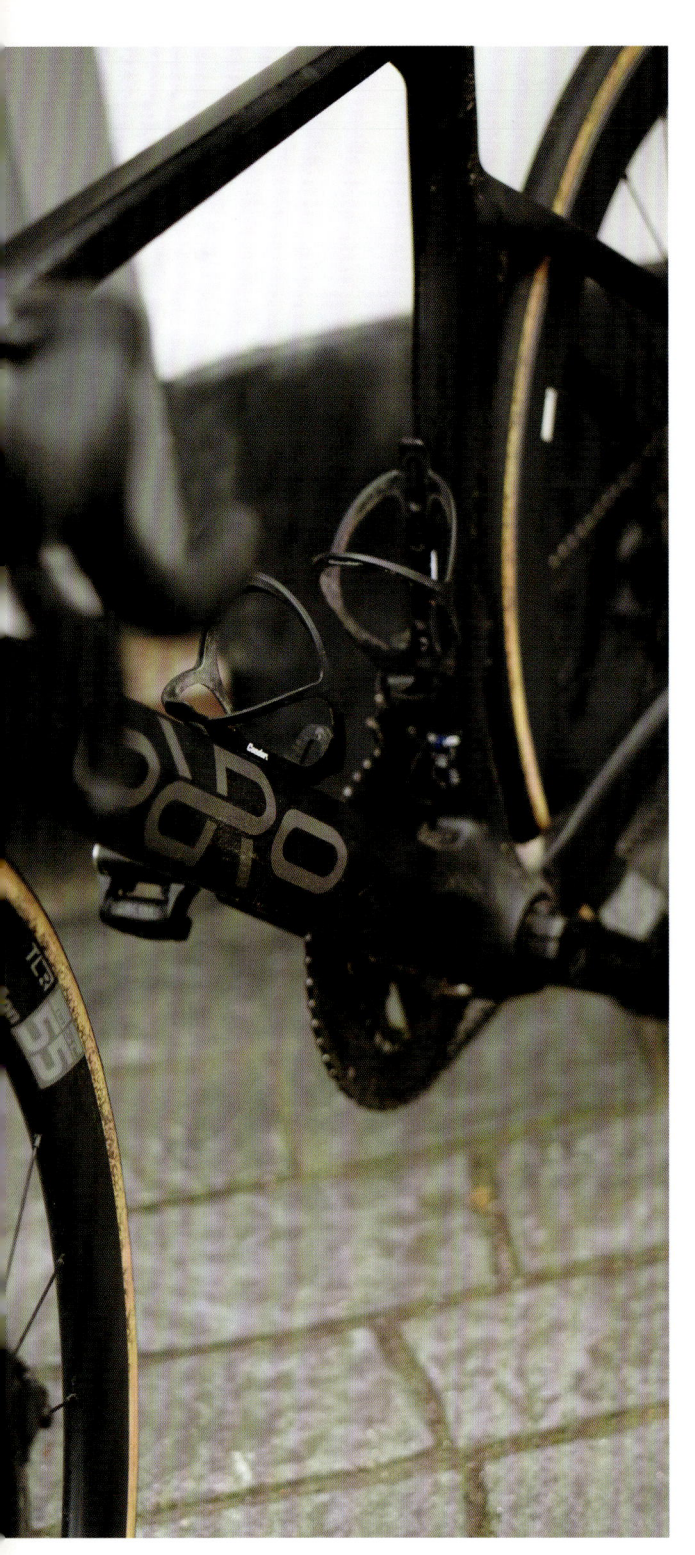

style unsuited to your natural position. Personally, I like to position my feet as near to the crank as possible without them actually touching.

Cranks

The crank affects your ability to generate force on the pedal and your comfort on the bike, so is worth consideration. I'm very much in the school of thought that cranks, which come as standard according to frame size (170–175mm/6.7–6.9in), are too long. Long cranks are not a problem in themselves, but there is little to be lost and much to be gained by opting for shorter cranks. Although the changes in power generated as a result of this are negligible, the advantages are in body position. Even just reducing the crank length by 5mm (0.2in) will not only provide a more comfortable aero position, but will keep your hip angle open, because your pedal stroke doesn't go too high. It also gives you better clearance when cornering. I'm 1.85m (6ft 1in) tall and ride with a 165mm (6.5in) crank, and I have no problems – I could even go smaller again.

Legs

There are many good reasons, aside from vanity, for having smooth legs as a cyclist. Being hairless is a lot better for massage and physio work, and also makes it much easier and less painful to take off plasters after crashes. What's more, I've done enough wind tunnel work to say confidently that shaving your legs means you'll also be a few watts and a second or two to the good. Free speed!

There are many good reasons, aside from vanity, for having smooth legs as a cyclist.

Clothing
Having sorted your positioning, apart from shaving your legs and washing your bike, wearing the correct clothing can be the best aero value for money. A modest outlay to upgrade your wardrobe can help you gain more than a few seconds, and they all add up!

Skinsuit
It might feel odd at first, like you are riding naked, but a well-fitting skinsuit can reduce your overall drag by as much as 10 per cent. As well as a streamlined surface, many include strategically placed aero strips or dimpled surfaces to increase airflow and minimise turbulence. They are available off-the-peg and if they fit tightly, they will almost certainly save you some time. It might not be much, though. Suits are specific, not only to cycling disciplines, but to individuals. The only real way to know if it is effective is to test it in a wind tunnel or do aero testing in a controlled environment such as an indoor track, although of course those aren't necessarily options for everyone.

Helmet
In terms of increased performance per pound, aero helmets maybe offer the best value. They can save you 20 seconds or more versus a non-aero helmet over a 40km (25-mile) ride and only cost £100 ($125) or so. In the past, traditional ventilated helmets were heavy on the drag, while aero helmets were unventilated and useless if you didn't keep your head raised. Now, road aero helmets have strategically placed vents (some can even be closed on colder days) and are designed so that looking down or to the side doesn't compromise their efficiency.

Shoes, covers and socks
At this point we are on to pretty marginal gains. Carbon-soled and sleekly designed aero shoes can make a small difference, although I've always found laces are more aero than boas. At most levels though, for a small outlay, shoe covers will be perfectly adequate. They smooth the airflow around your lower leg and reduce the friction of buckles and laces. Socks made with special aero fabric and design are about the cheapest modification you can make and even if they don't actually make a huge difference, they might make you *feel* faster, which is part of the battle.

FLEXIBILITY

Lexie Williamson

Toe-touching may be a challenge and your Lotus pose days a distant memory, but there are still big benefits to be had by investing in flexibility work as a midlife cyclist. Simply sitting on the saddle will be a lot more comfortable and there may even be aero gains. So, to that end, here are the bare stretching essentials to stave off stiffness.

How flexible does a midlife cyclist need to be?

Short answer: you don't need to be a gymnast. Avoid aggressive, deep stretches that push you beyond your natural range. It's not necessary to sweat buckets in hot yoga or tie yourself in knots (unless that's your thing). It genuinely doesn't matter if you can't touch your toes or sit cross-legged. Honestly, no one cares.

It does matter, however, if an increasingly stiff body is affecting comfort levels in the saddle. Maybe you've cut a long ride short due to lower back ache or have a dull, persistent ache in the back of the neck. Provided these are not bike fit issues, they can often be easily remedied with a little regular strength and mobility work.

So, what should you be doing if you have so far resisted adopting a stretching routine? The good news is that there's a lot you don't have to do. Downward Dog, for example, will feature heavily in many yoga videos but holding Dog pose makes little sense for the cyclist who probably already has tension-laden shoulders. You can also probably omit yoga's balances if your legs feel tired and heavy.

The trick for cyclists is to focus on a few key spots like the hip flexors, hamstrings, lower back, glutes and quads, and any yoga positions that flip the hunched-over riding position into reverse, such as gentle back bends and lunges.

If you feel tight before you ride it's useful to loosen up, especially if you've been chained to the desk all day, and there are a few simple mobility routines that will warm you up pre-ride in this chapter.

But what you *really* need to do to improve your overall flexibility (and this might not be popular with the endorphin junkies) is to sit still. Yes, it takes a bit of patience, but it's time well spent. Research shows that it you want to improve flexibility you need to hold a stretch. The sports science world is still arguing over exactly how long to hold, but 20 seconds should cover it. Let's delve into some techniques to stay nice and bendy.

The science of stretching

'But stretching is so boring!' Yes, yes, I know, but a little dedication will reap rewards, I promise. Unfortunately, for the fidgety cycling types, holding a stretch stock still is the key to improving flexibility. Wrapped around the muscle fibres are muscle 'spindles' and it's their job to tell the muscle to contract if they sense they might be in danger of overstretching (and therefore being damaged). If we enter the stretch slowly and then hold still, this will override the signal and the muscle then relaxes. This static stretching should be accompanied by slow, deep breathing, as this triggers the 'rest-and-relax' or parasympathetic side of the nervous system, which further encourages muscle release.

Stretching and power reduction

The thinking in the sports science world is to save the static stretching (moving a muscle to a point of tension and holding still) for after your ride, as a number of studies have found that it temporarily reduces the power output of muscles. Opt instead for dynamic, or moving, techniques as shown below to warm up and improve mobility. After the ride your muscles will welcome a nice deep stretch, especially if accompanied by slow, deep breathing.

Stretching: why should I bother?

Good question. Cycling does not require you to lunge sideways to kick a ball or reach overhead for that tennis serve. Just the opposite: you barely move for three hours. But therein lies the reason for a little bit of loosening up. It's partly so we can happily hold this position and partly so we can break out of it and function as a human being the rest of the time. Keeping particularly the back and hips supple has a performance benefit for cyclists, too, in terms of helping to achieve a more aero position. But mostly it's about comfort and just riding for as long as your heart desires.

Flexibility matters if an increasingly stiff body is affecting comfort levels in the saddle.

Post-ride stretches

Instead of lots of yoga exercises (for a wide range of sequences, try *Yoga for Cyclists*), here's just one brief routine for the reluctant stretcher. This six-step sequence hits all the cycling tight spots with minimum fuss. Supplement with the add-ons (*see* p.66) if you want a longer routine.

1) LYING TWIST

Lie on your back with your legs bent and your feet flat on the floor and together. Position your arms out to the sides in line with your shoulders. Drop both knees to the right.

Hold for 20 seconds, then repeat on the other side.

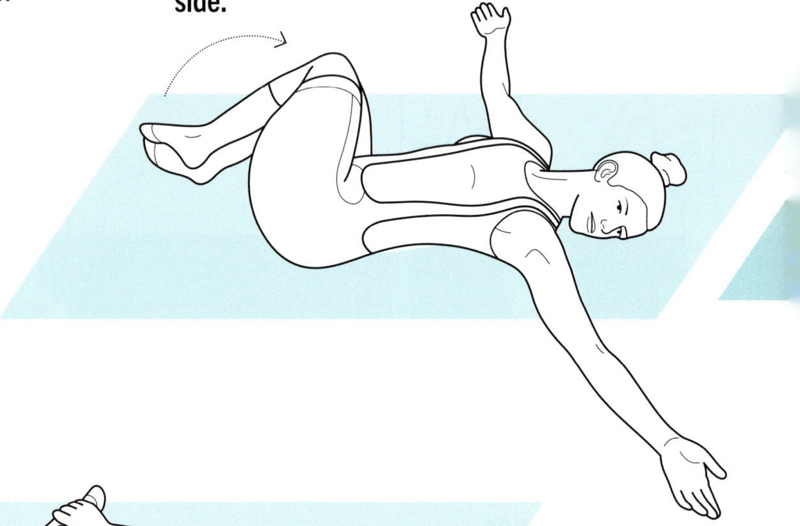

2) PRONE QUAD STRETCH

Lie on your front. Bend your left leg and reach around to grab the left foot with your left hand. Press your hips into the floor and slowly draw your foot closer to the body.

Hold for 20 seconds, then switch legs.

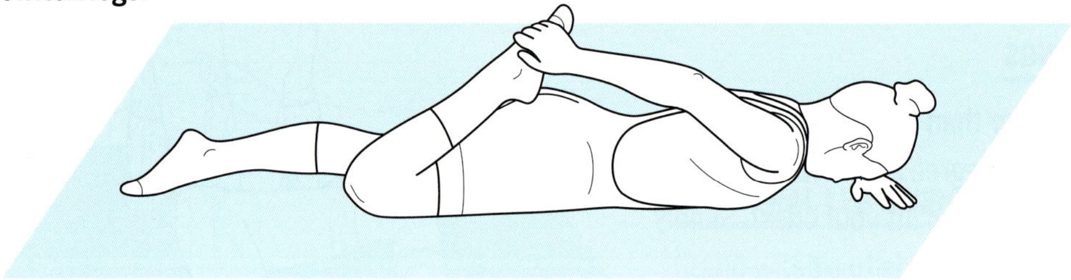

3) PUPPY DOG

From all fours, walk your hands above your head along the floor and sink your chest towards the floor. Your knees should remain under your hips.

Hold for 20 seconds.

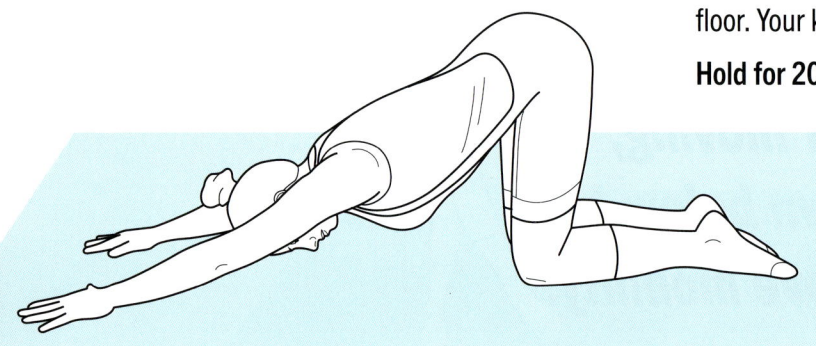

FLEXIBILITY

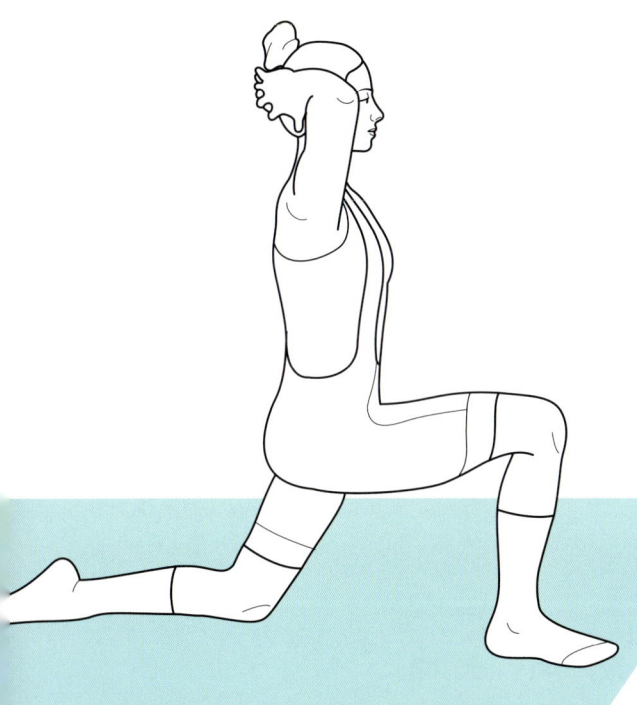

4) LOW LUNGE

From all fours, step your right foot up in between your hands and lift your upper body. Tuck your backside in and take your hands behind your head. Slide slowly forwards into the lunge (this can be done standing if it's uncomfortable to kneel).

Hold for 20 seconds, then switch sides.

5) FIGURE-FOUR

Lie on your back with your legs bent. Place your left ankle on top of your right thigh and flex your left foot. Now hug both legs in towards you, holding them either behind your right thigh or just below your right knee.

Hold for 20 seconds, then switch sides.

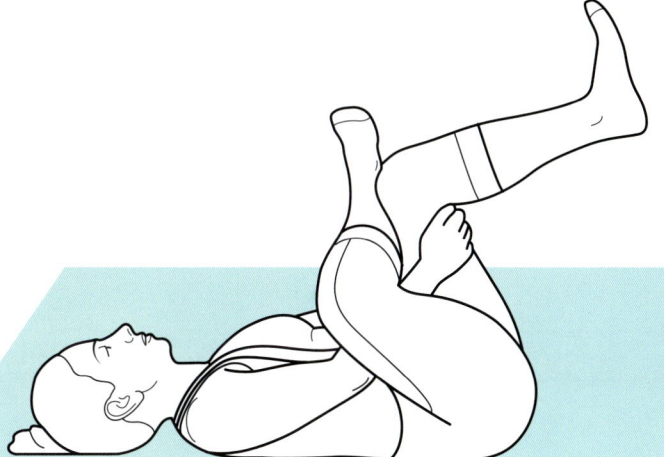

If you only do one stretch today...

...make it figure-four. Most of us are familiar with that pain in the middle of the backside; the bit the massage therapist leans their elbow into, causing you to utter a few choice swear words. The beauty of this stretch is that it can be done lying, sitting on the floor, or even sitting at your desk in a meeting. Sit on a chair with a straight back and place your right heel on your left thigh. Maintaining a straight spine, lean forwards until you feel a stretch in the butt.

FULL GAS FOREVER

6) HAMSTRING STRAP STRETCH

Lie on your back with your legs out straight. Bend your right knee and loop a strap, tie or jumper sleeve around your right foot. Straighten your right leg up towards the ceiling if you can, but keep a bend in the leg if the hamstring feels tight.

Hold for 20 seconds, then switch legs.

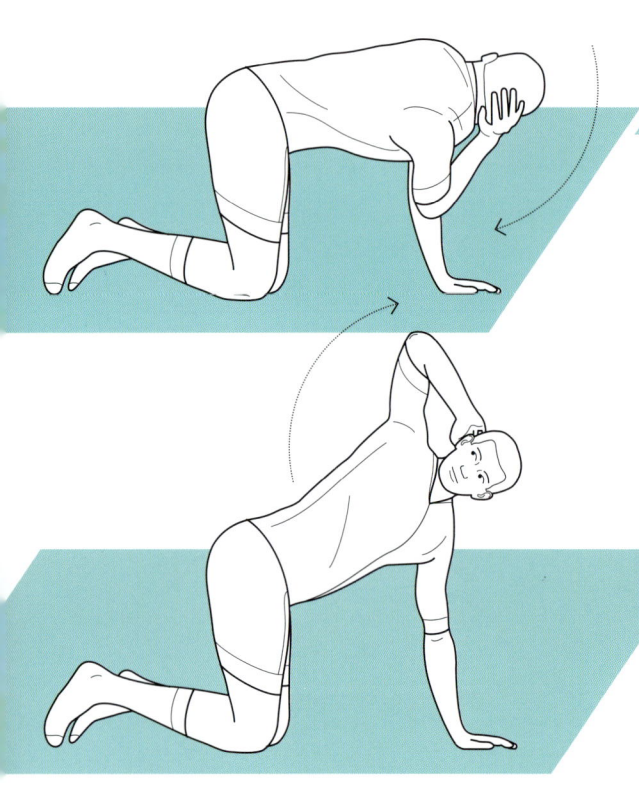

All fours add-ons

Add these after Puppy Dog if you want a longer sequence.

1) THORACIC TWIST

Position your knees a bit wider in all fours. Place your right fingertips on your right ear. Keep looking down. As you inhale, point your elbow up to the ceiling, and as you exhale, point it down.

Repeat three more times, then switch sides.

2) KNEELING LAT STRETCH

From all fours, take your knees wide and your big toes close. Sit slowly back into a frog-leg position and stretch your arms overhead on the floor. Crawl your hands round to the right, place your left hand on top of your right one and interlace your fingers.

Hold for 10 seconds, then switch sides.

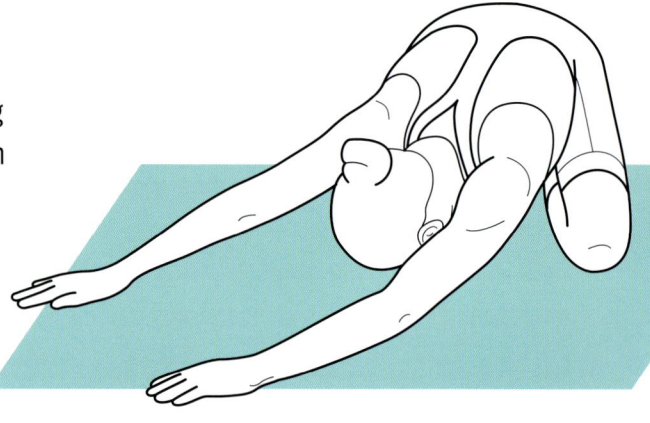

Standing add-ons

Add these after low lunge if you want a longer sequence.

1) TRIANGLE

Stand up from your lunge and step your feet wide apart. Turn your right foot out 90 degrees and your left foot in 45 degrees. Raise your arms up to shoulder height. Lean to your right and rest your right hand on your thigh or lower leg. Reach your left arm up to the ceiling or over by your left ear.

Hold for 20 seconds, then switch sides.

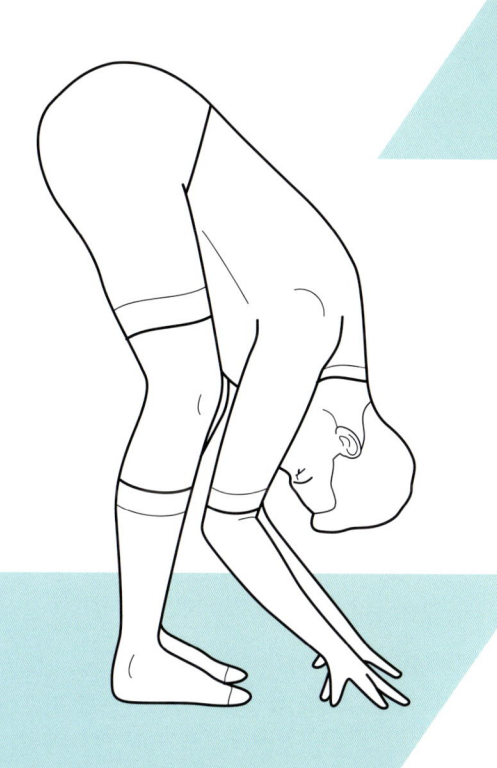

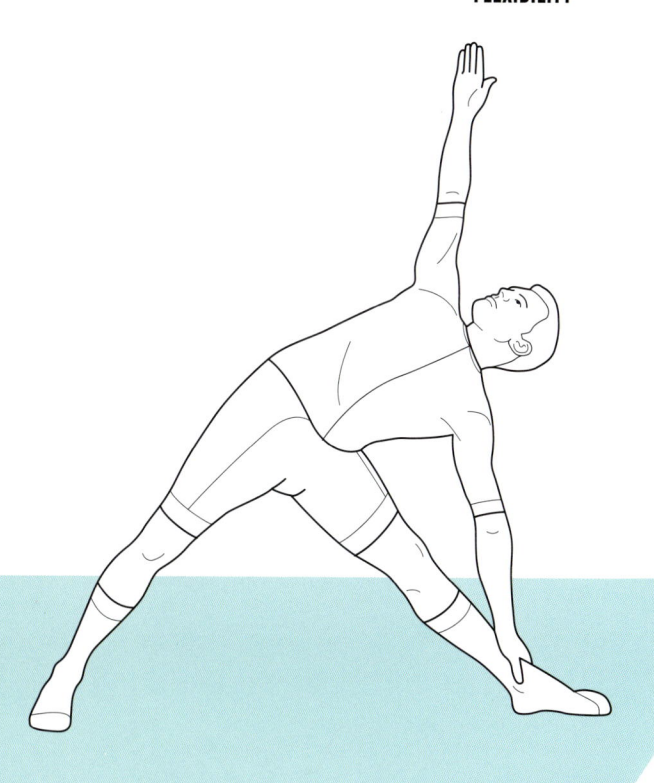

2) HAMSTRING HANG

Stand with your legs wide apart and turn your toes slightly inwards. Place your hands on your hips and tip forwards. Either rest your hands on your thighs or place them on the floor. Relax your head.

Hold for 20 seconds, then rise up with a straight back and your core engaged.

FULL GAS FOREVER

Three stretches for the stiffest cyclist

Flexibility-challenged? Here are four stretches for even the stiffest rider. You'll need a cotton yoga strap or just use an old tie or rolled-up towel for exercises 1 and 4. Anyone can do these! So, no excuses.

1) THE W

To stretch your chest muscles and shoulders after being crunched over the handlebars, simply stand or sit up straight, hold the strap taut between your hands, then bring it overhead and bend your arms into a W shape. Draw your arms back to increase the intensity.

Hold for 20 seconds.

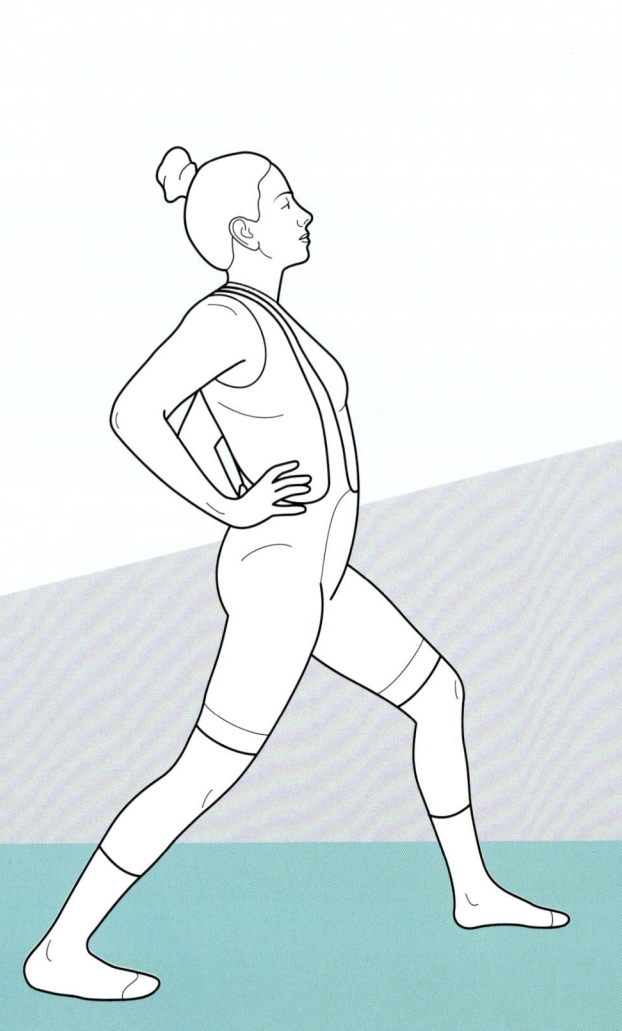

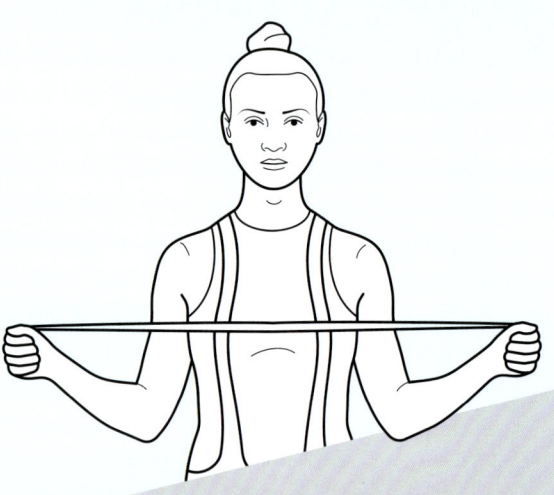

2) STANDING LUNGE

Step one leg back and bend the front leg. Tuck your backside in and place your hands on your hips or hook your thumbs behind your back.

Hold for 20 seconds, then switch sides.

The best hip flexor stretch is probably done kneeling.

3) 90-DEGREE LONG ROLLER/WALL STRETCH

Place your hands on the roller or wall surface and walk backwards until your body forms a 90-degree angle. Hold and breathe slowly here, thinking about sinking the chest down or leaning slightly away from your hands to increase the stretch.

Hold for 20 seconds.

Find your hip flexors

There's one golden rule with stretching the front of your hips and that's 'tuck your backside in'. The best hip flexor stretch is probably done kneeling. Come into a tall kneeling position (put a cushion under your knee if it's uncomfortable), then step one leg forward and put your hands on your hips. Keeping your backside tucked in, slide slowly into the lunge. Hold for a good 20 seconds, breathing slowly, then switch sides.

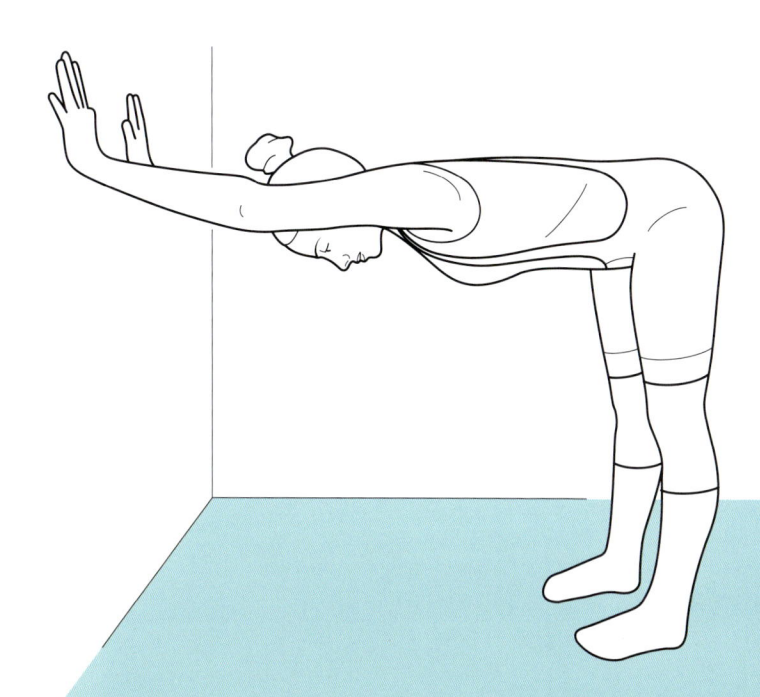

FULL GAS FOREVER

Four moves for a happy back

A happy back is a mobile back. Backs need to be stretched or moved through different planes of motion: flexion, extension, lateral flexion and rotation (aka leaning forwards, back, to the side and then twisting movements). Work through these and your back will thank you.

1) SEATED TWIST

Sit on the floor with your legs straight. Step your right leg over your left. Wrap your left arm around your right knee. Place your right hand behind you and rotate your torso to the right.

Hold for 10 seconds, then switch sides.

2) LATERAL FLEXION

Standing, raise your right arm up and side bend to the left, sliding your left hand down your left thigh. Try not to lean forwards or back.

Hold for a few seconds, then repeat to the right side. Repeat four times on each side.

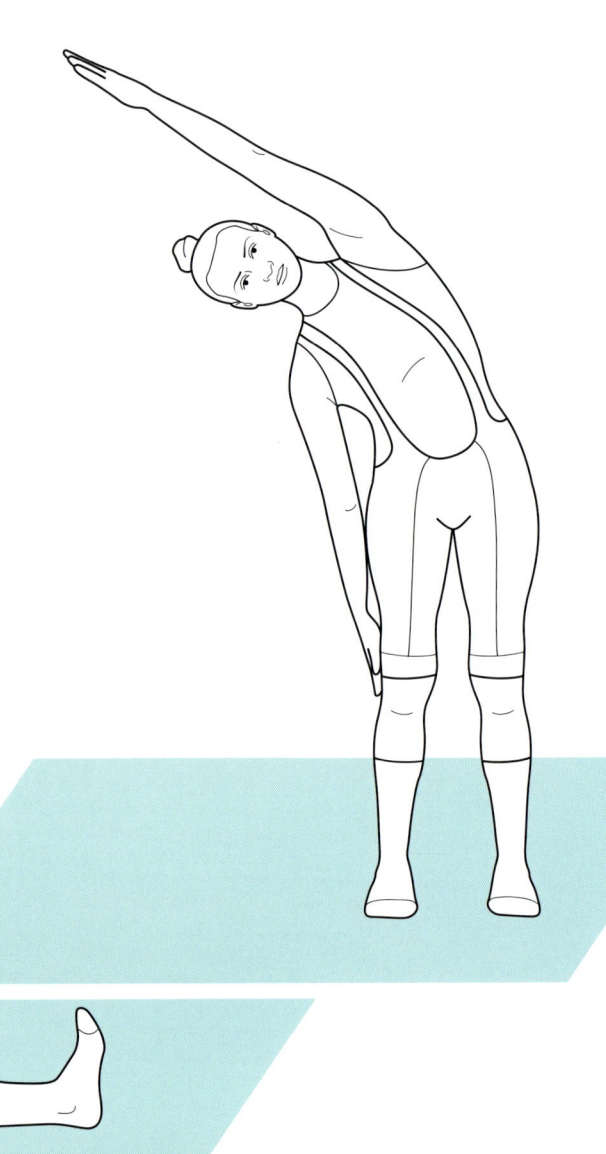

3) SPINAL EXTENSION

From standing or tall kneeling, place your palms on your lower back and move into a gentle backbend.

Hold for 5–10 seconds, then rise up.

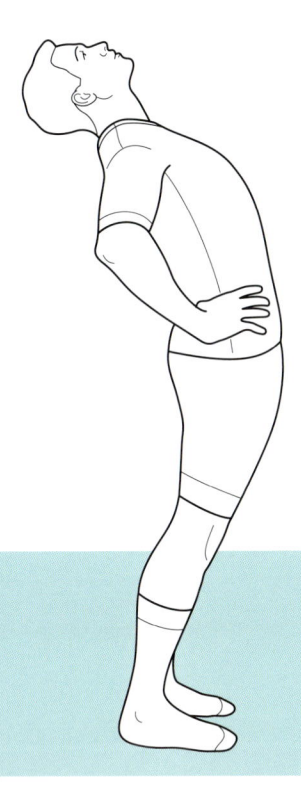

Backs need to be stretched or moved through different planes of motion: flexion, extension, lateral flexion and rotation.

4) SPINAL FLEXION

Standing, bend your knees and fold forwards, allowing your back to round and your head to relax. Fold your arms or let them dangle.

Hold for 10 seconds. To rise up safely, bend your knees, straighten your back and engage your core.

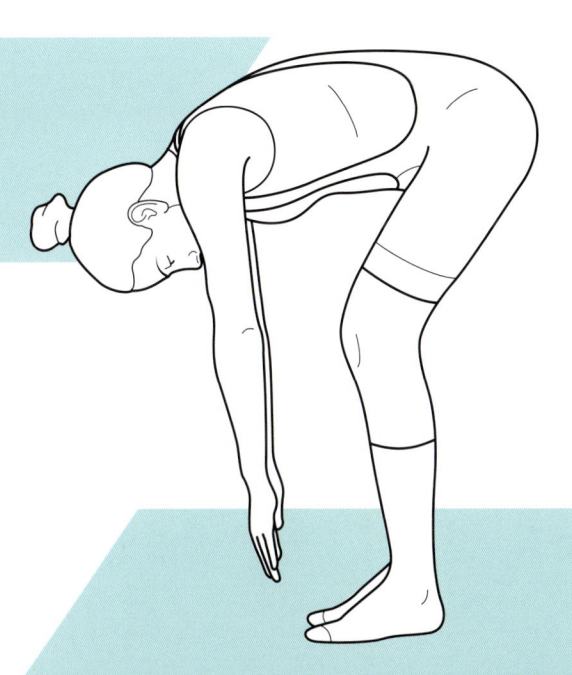

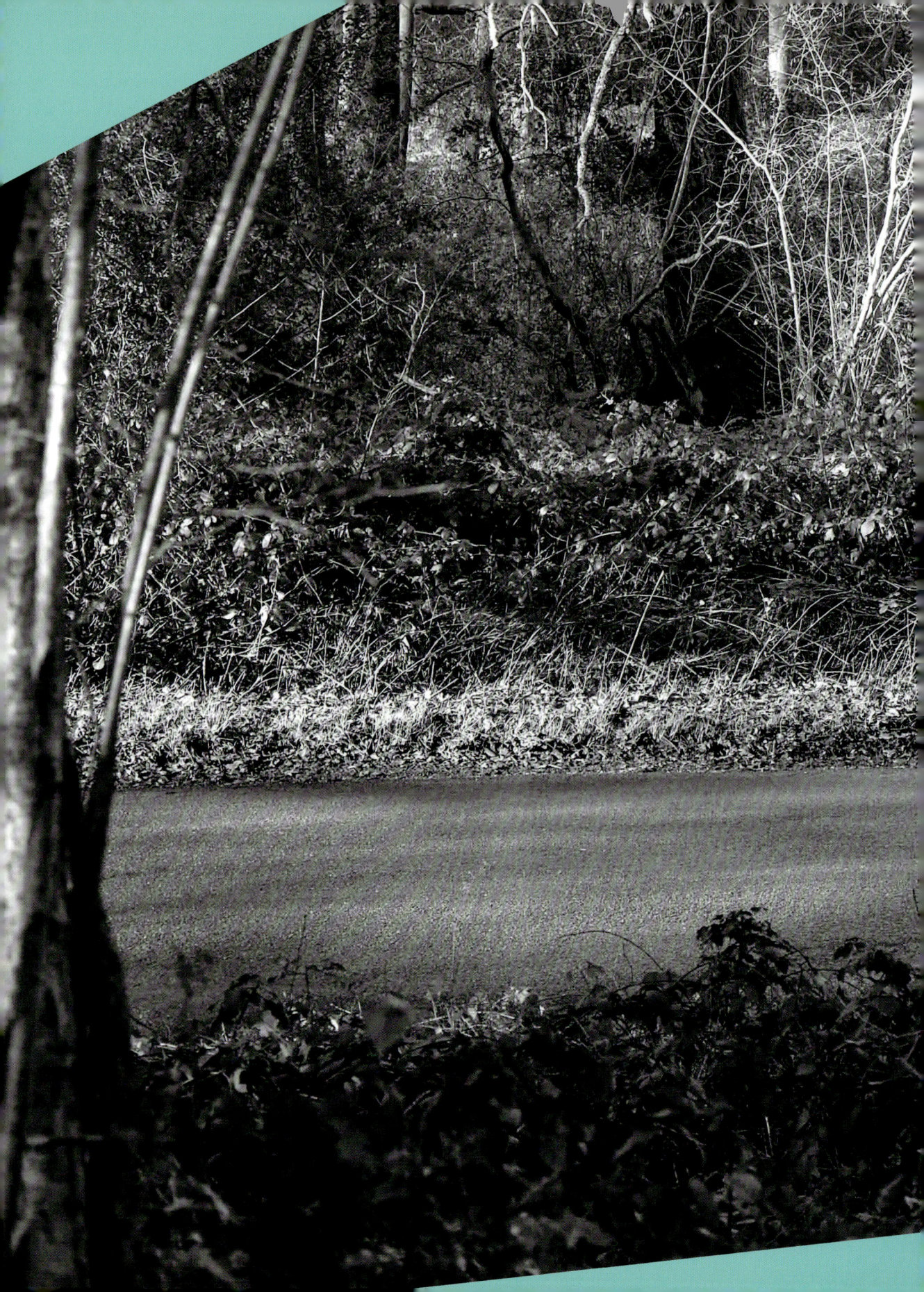

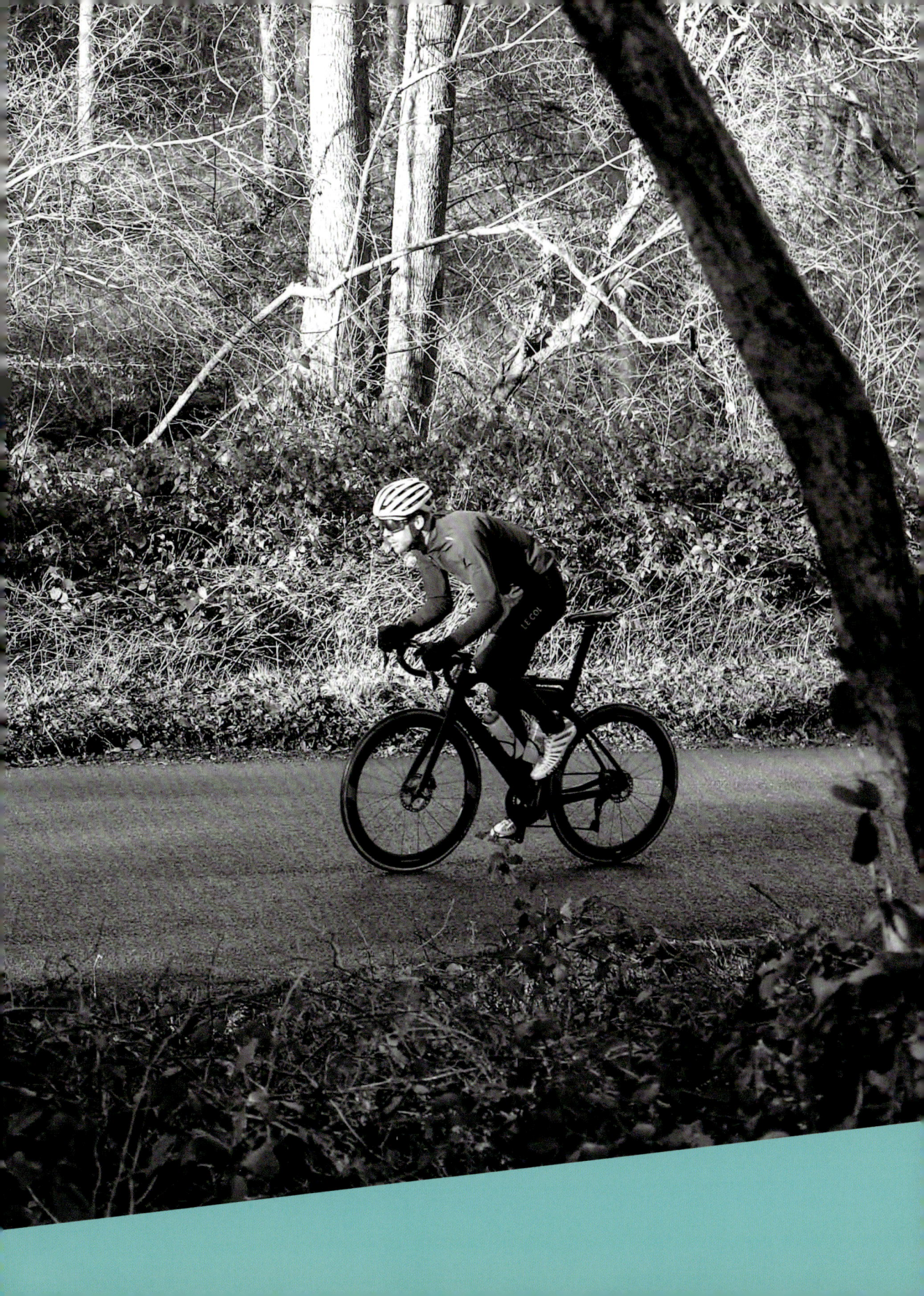

NIGGLES

Lexie Williamson

Two hours into the club ride and, yep, there it is again . . . that sensation in the left butt cheek. It's not painful enough to stop the ride, but is distracting you from the views, the sunshine and the chat. Yes, most of us will have our fair share of niggles, but treating a potential injury early on can keep you off the sofa and on the road, where you belong.

Stop procrastinating and 'get it seen soon'

This chapter explores how to prevent, spot and treat some of the classic cycling niggles, with help from a few of our cycling-specialist physio friends. We're not talking about broken collar bones here, but those annoying wear-and-tear issues caused by the repetitive nature of cycling. You can get away with it for years and then, there it is again, that left butt cheek complaining on every pedal stroke.

First off, it's tempting to ignore these sorts of niggles and hope they'll go away, but the mantra from the experts is 'get it seen soon'. The solution is probably quick and simple. 'Often niggles can be fixed with a tweak to your bike fit or a new saddle, and you can return to training as long and hard as your training plan dictates,' says Phil Cavell, author of *The Midlife Cyclist* and cycling biomechanics expert/bike fitter extraordinaire.

Cavell puts most injuries down to an 'information and moderation deficit'. For example, foot pain arises because an athlete's shoe wasn't chosen to suit their foot type. Back, neck and shoulder pain appear due to incorrect positioning and posture on the bike. 'If a problem is tackled early on during its acute phase, removal of the underlying cause is enough to instantly deal with the pain, and the problem goes away. If a rider ignores the issue it's likely to become chronic and the affected tissues and structures are now damaged,' Cavell says.

If you are lucky enough to live near a cycling-specialist physio, hunt them down, as trying to run an internet search on causes of common riding overuse injuries will take you down a rabbit hole and there's no substitute for an experienced pair of eyes. But also, a physio who 'gets' cycling will totally understand why riding 90km (55 miles) every Sunday is a perfectly normal thing to want to do and will work hard to keep you attending those rides.

NIGGLES

Treating a potential injury early on can keep you off the sofa and on the road, where you belong.

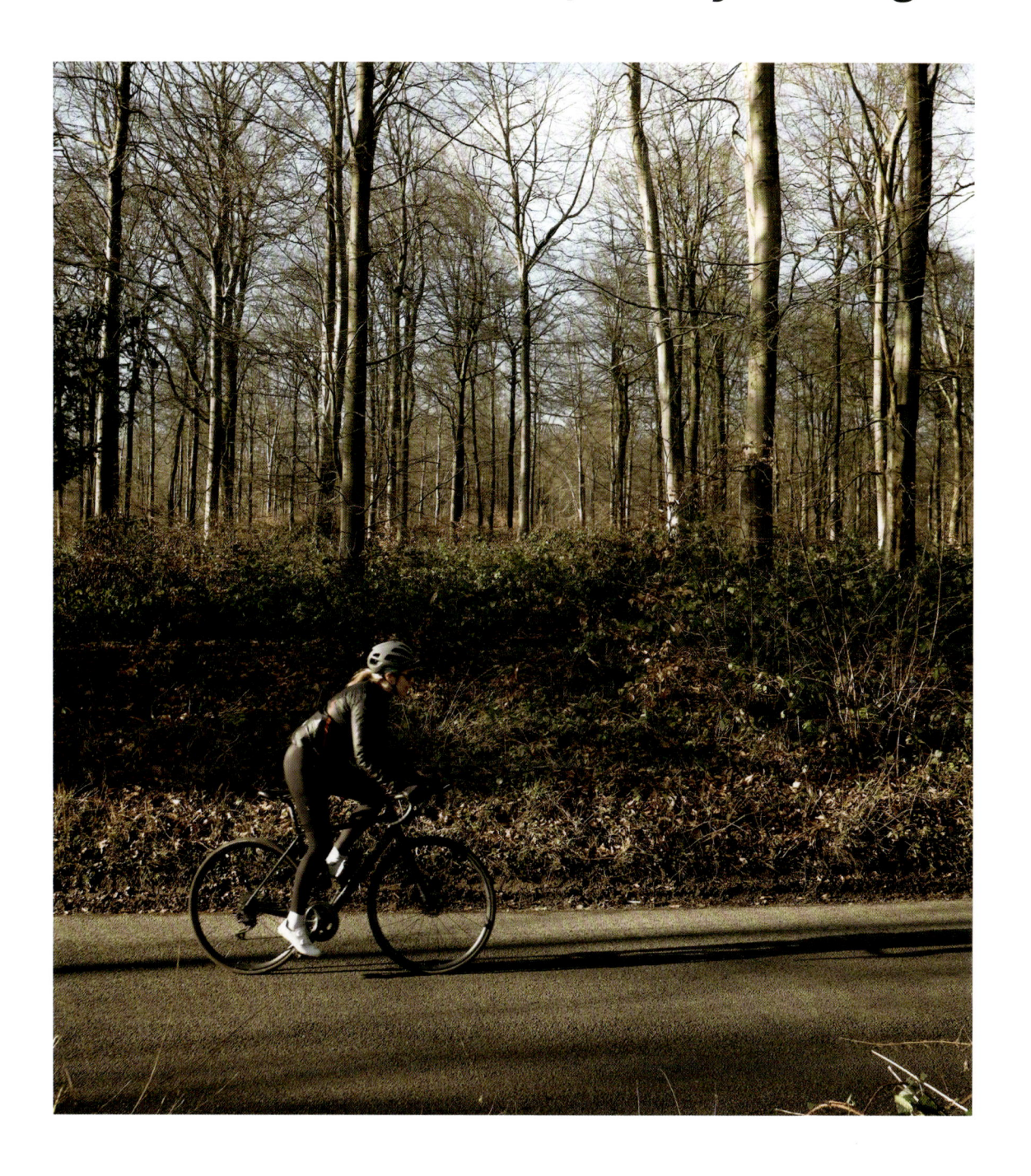

FULL GAS FOREVER

We have sought out three such specialist physio superstars and quizzed them about the most common areas we complain to them about.

Hip pain
Signs and symptoms

'Hip problems can manifest in a few ways,' says Bianca Broadbent, the first of our gurus. 'One manifestation might be a loss of range of motion. This might not be obvious initially, but you may notice that you can't lift your leg to step over the bike frame. Or maybe you can't bring your hip through the full range on the pedal stroke; you're sitting asymmetrically (leaning more to one side) or are pedalling with your knees out.'

According to Broadbent you may also develop pain in the hip itself, or the knee. The latter is known as 'referred pain'. Hip pain usually manifests as a positive 'c sign'. The name comes from patients making a pincer grip around their hips with the thumb and forefinger when asked, 'Where does it hurt?' The causes of this pain could stem from a number of things, including osteoarthritis of the hip, issues with the labrum (the specialised cartilage that surrounds the hip socket) such as a tear, or an 'FAI' or femoroacetabular impingement of the hip. This is where the ball and socket meet awkwardly, causing a bony 'impingement'. Or it might be due to a combination of the above.

Prehab tips
- Get another bike fit. Most of us only have a bike fit once, but Broadbent explains that the bike position you were in 5–10 years ago may not be optimal now, and these conditions are aggravated by trying to cycle with a range of movement incompatible with your current anatomy.
- Troubleshoot to improve your bike fit by making tweaks in small, reversible increments just to see if they work for you.
- Try switching to shorter cranks, raising the cockpit and checking the saddle height.
- Take up strength training – something that all our gurus advocate (*see* chapter 3).

'There are a number of treatments depending on the diagnosis,' says Broadbent. But for some, the only route for hip issues is surgery. That might mean hip resurfacing or a complete hip replacement. On a more positive note, she believes that as long as the bike set-up doesn't demand too much hip flexion from the rider, cycling can actually be beneficial for these conditions as it is a low-contact sport.

Lower back pain
Signs and symptoms
It doesn't require a physiotherapy degree to see that spending hours with a hunched-over back could, um . . . lead to back issues. Not many riders get away without the odd niggle here. But Broadbent warns against automatically assuming an association between the flexed riding posture and pain. She also notes the difference between treating lower back pain that exists in everyday life, but is aggravated by cycling, and lower back pain that is purely cycling driven, as the two are very different.

Get your bike position checked by a professional fitter. Also, consider the amount of time you spend in this position and the kind of riding you are planning; one position might be perfectly suited to short, hard crits, but become a lower back nightmare on a multi-day stage race.

Finally, lower back ache could be traced to a lack of muscular endurance, particularly in the core and hips, which means the back becomes overloaded when the legs tire. Lower back problems also often occur in new riders who have yet to develop sufficient leg strength or who overtrain and under-recover (do too many hard rides).

Prehab tips
- Offload acute episodes of lower back pain with active recovery. This might be gentle movement such as walking, Pilates or yoga. Consider your flexibility and then see if your bike position matches that level.
- Change your bike position depending on the type of riding you plan to do and seek help from a physio and bike fitter to trace the root cause.
- Check your saddle isn't positioned too high or too far back. Also check it isn't too narrow and is supportive enough.
- Ensure your cockpit is not too high, low, close or far away.
- Check your cranks are not too long.

Get another bike fit. The bike position you were in 10 years ago may not be optimal now.

Buttock pain
Signs and symptoms

If you have a niggling pain in the backside there are a couple of key sources to consider that may be driving your pain, says cycling specialist physio and bike fitter Bryan McCullough.

- **The hip joint** – 'In our 20–30s a common diagnosis here may be some form of hip impingement. As we age, we have an increasing chance of age-related joint problems such as osteoarthritis becoming symptomatic [painful]. This can either cause pain at the front of the hip and groin crease, refer pain deeper into the buttock area, or even down the thigh. If you have buttock pain and have noticed that the hip joint on this side is stiffer to move, or has more limited range of movement, especially first thing in the morning, it is worth discussing this with your GP, who may be able to arrange a hip X-ray.'
- **The lumbar spine (lower back)** – 'For the same reasons as above it can become more common to have some degree of change at the joints in the lower spine or indeed some narrowing of the intervertebral discs. With narrower discs or some inflammation around the facet joints there is an increased possibility of irritation of the nerve roots that exit the spine. This can lead to a variety of pains that could manifest as buttock ache, sharp pain down the back of the thigh or sciatica where the pain can radiate all the way down the leg (a burning or tingling sensation).'

Prehab tips

- Improve your hip mobility; yoga is a fantastic way to do this.
- Strength exercises are the cornerstone to hip health. Even bodyweight exercises such as squats, glute bridges and side steps with a band around your ankles are a great starting point.
- Check your saddle height. Too high and it will increase the likelihood of overreaching. This leads to both a sore lower back and creates instability in the pelvis, which forces the buttock muscles to work overtime in order to regain stability.
- Check your handlebars are not too far away or too low. This forces the rider into a more flexed position, closing down the hip angle and increasing the chance of buttock pain and hip impingement.
- Check your crank length. Consider the height of the pedalling circle at the 12 o' clock position. 'If you find it hard to bring the knee to the chest off the bike it's likely that you'll find a shorter crank easier to manage on the bike,' explains McCullough.

Essentially, the overriding message regarding bike fit is to minimise unnecessary hip movement when riding, because it creates instability on the saddle, which can lead to buttock pain.

Neck tension
Signs and symptoms

Localised tension around the neck and shoulders during riding may arise from overloaded muscles, which leads to muscular tension, but could also indicate underlying issues at the neck joints or discs.

- **Muscular tension** – This is the most common reason for developing aching around the upper shoulder and neck area, says McCullough. The muscles here work hard in a fixed position, often for a long duration, which leads to tissue overload. This often manifests as a dull, nagging ache around the base of the neck/top of the shoulders.
- **Neck joints** – While cycling, we hold our heads in an extended position (torso forwards and head up). This essentially requires the joints to close down to the end of their range, which can become painful or limited (or both) if there are joint-related changes such as osteoarthritis.
- **Neck discs** – As we age, our intervertebral discs will tend to be more dehydrated and, as a result, become narrower. This reduces the spaces for the nerves to exit from the spine. The discs also become less flexible, so we may suffer with a 'strain' to the disc, or a disc bulge. Both are painful in their own right, but can also irritate the nerve roots, which leads to severe pain, tingling or numbness that radiates down the arm to the fingers.

Prehab tips

- Maximise flexibility through all the neck joints and surrounding muscles by moving your neck through its full range of motion. Try yoga but never push into pain.
- Work on upper back mobility, too – it's crucial. The better your mid- and upper back move, the less your neck has to compensate to hold a good position while riding. Try the Thoracic Twist exercise, found on page 68, or place a foam roller underneath the thoracic (mid) spine and lean back to move the spine into extension.
- Consider neck strengthening exercises. For example, lie on your back and tuck in your chin to make a slight double chin. Then lift the head an inch off the floor and hold here, maintaining the chin tuck. Men should be able to hold this position for 39 seconds and women for 29 seconds.
- Have a regular massage to loosen tension, improve circulation and ease pain.
- Avoid setting up your bike with excessive reach or drop to the front of the bike. Reducing the reach and raising the front end can make a big difference.
- Handlebars that are too wide for your shoulders can often increase shoulder/neck tension.
- Ensure you are not leaning heavily on the handlebars, as you will more likely lock out your arms, which leads to tension around the neck caused by vibration from the road.

Lateral knee pain
Signs and symptoms
Lateral knee pain often occurs when the iliotibial band (ITB) tendon is irritated by compression and/or rubbing during cycling, says Dr Graham Theobald, a physio with a doctorate in cycling-related knee pain. Initially you might feel pain on every pedal stroke. If it becomes hot, inflamed or swollen, see a clinician as soon as possible. Theobald warns that with lateral knee pain the cause might actually be further up the chain of muscles, such as tight and weak glutes and abductors (outer thigh muscles).

'Keep a constant eye on these areas because as you get older, things change. Muscles weaken as part of the normal ageing process, so maintaining strength and conditioning becomes super important,' he adds.

Prehab tips
- Strengthen the gluteus maximus and gluteus medius (side of the hip) and the abductors (side of the thigh) as well as the tensor fasciae latae muscle on the outer hip.
- Check your saddle isn't too high, causing ITB compression.
- Check your saddle isn't too far forward or back, resulting in excessive knee loading.
- Check whether you have a leg length discrepancy, which causes an imbalance and reduces the power you drive through the knee on indoor trainers.

Anterior knee pain
Signs and symptoms
Are you experiencing soreness under the kneecap or just below? It could be patellar tendonitis (inflammation or the tendon) if the pain increases during the ride. Anterior knee pain also worsens with higher loads – for example, pushing through a higher gear – and is often relieved by standing in the saddle when climbing, as this shifts some of the work away from the quads and to muscles like the glutes. 'Older cyclists often experience degeneration of the cartilage on the underside of the kneecap, which requires effective management,' explains Theobald.

Prehab tips
- Check whether your seat is too low or far forwards. If either is the case, you may be creating excessive knee force.
- Overly long cranks can also result in too much torque through the pedal stroke.
- Try moving your cleats further back if they are set forward. Strengthen all muscle groups, not just the quads and glutes.
- Keep your knees warm and focus on smooth, efficient pedalling rather than erratic surging.
- Consider a more endurance-based bike geometry, as the angles developed in their design reduce shock loads on the joints.

Knee niggles and the indoor trainer

'As midlife riders we're told one of the main routes to sustaining VO_2 max and maintaining muscle mass is short, sharp interval training sessions. But the way some use indoor trainers to do these sessions puts their knees under excessive pressure,' states Theobald. 'I still see some coaches advocating low cadence/high resistance and some older riders are doing these kind of old-school sessions frequently.'

He adds: 'Degeneration of a joint is normal as we age; the tendons become brittle, we develop thinner menisci through wear and tear and cartilage breaks down. Therefore, these sessions can really take their toll on your body. Your body needs a little respect as you get older. It is possible to achieve high power numbers with a higher cadence. Finding the highest cadence alongside the most sustainable heart rate/power is key to developing as a 50-plus cyclist. Shorter cranks can assist a higher cadence so also consider this.'

Training apps like Zwift can also create the pressure to deliver explosive, seated power sessions where riders are driving through the knee.

'These riders are also not moving or changing position as they would naturally be when riding on the road,' says Theobald. This, combined with the competition pressures of riding with others, where everyone can see your watts on screen, means indoor training can be brutal on the knees. 'Men are worse; the egos get in the way and they do too much, too hard.'

Is it a niggle or an injury?

On the pain scale, with 1 being pain-free and 10 being a career-ending injury, a niggle is somewhere in the middle; it hurts but generally not enough to prevent you from riding. If you feel the niggle on every ride as the miles mount up and over a period of a few weeks, get it checked out by a physio. Extreme discomfort or high levels of pain may indicate that a medical specialist and treatment are required.

Niggle prehab

All the physios in this chapter recommend working on strength and maintaining a good level of mobility as good prehab, or as preventative tactics for common riding niggles. On the mobility front, do gentle yoga or Pilates or walking as active recovery, especially for issues such as back pain. For strength, try squats, deadlifts, leg presses and side planks, and build up your core. Also, don't just work on the obvious glutes and quads, but remember to include the outside hip, calves and hamstrings. Bryan McCullough is a particular advocate of strength training, especially if you are riding a lot. 'You might be doing 5,000 pedal strokes an hour, but if your muscles are stronger, the effect of this on the body will be less.'

DOES MENTAL PERFORMANCE MATTER?

Ed Clancy

The mental aspect of cycling is just as important as the physical. Ensuring you are driven by your goals and make decisions based on facts is the basis of a high-performance mindset.

You look at top riders before a race. Some of them look stressed and anxious; others seem cool and unconcerned. But as soon as that race starts, they are switched on. If not, they've already lost. So much of cycling – training and racing – goes on in the head. Whatever discipline you are riding – road, track, mountain biking – your level of decision-making, confidence, motivation, application and pain management are as important as your physical fitness. The right mindset can ultimately be the difference between an average and an elite rider. So, how can you get your head space right?

The 'why'

You have to have a dream. A big dream. If it's big enough that people doubt you or think you are mad, then you are in the right ballpark. There's no point in choosing something easy. It has to be aspirational. You don't even have to tell people – it can be your secret – but think big. It has to be something that will get you out of bed. It has to be the *why*. If the why is strong enough, you get up and out on the bike on a rainy day, you put in that extra effort when your body wants to give up and you drink sparkling water when your mates are ordering lagers.

There are three levels of motivation in cycling. Everyone knows *what* they are doing. They are out regularly, riding fast and pushing themselves. Then there are those who are more involved in their sport and know *how* they are going about it; there's some plan of how they will make progress. Finally, there are those who can tell you *why* they

DOES MENTAL PERFORMANCE MATTER?

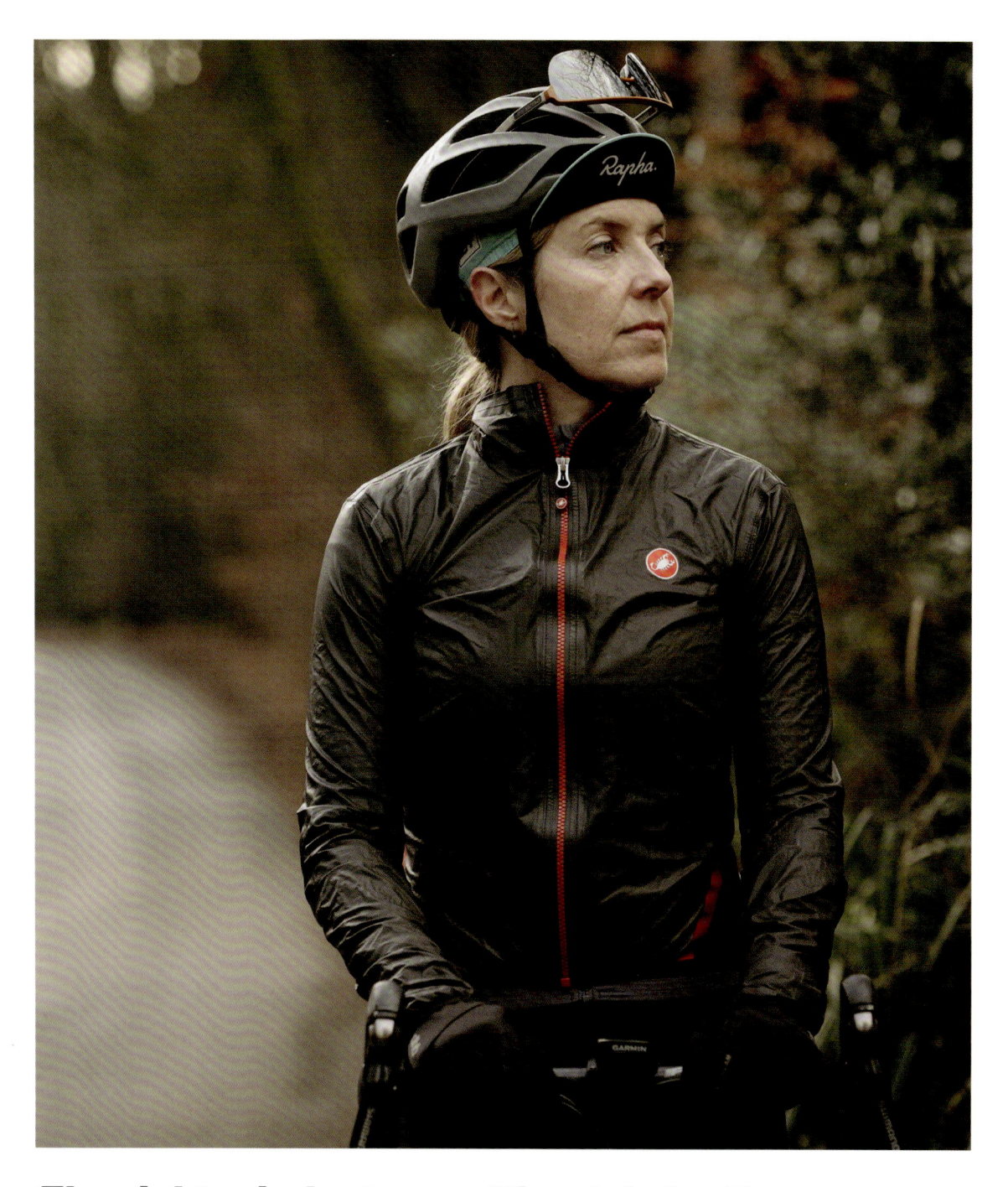

The right mindset can ultimately be the difference between an average and an elite rider.

are doing it. Why they have picked this sport. Why they are training or why they have entered this race. Those who have ready answers to these questions are the ones who really get it: the ones who have a purpose – a goal, a dream, a motivation. I'm going to win that sportive next year. I'm going to raise money for my mate's charity. I'm doing it for my family to be proud of me or I'm doing it to inspire a generation.

> After the Tour of Britain in 2015, I suffered a freak injury as I turned to pick up a suitcase. I was diagnosed with a prolapsed disc and was on anti-inflammatories and epidurals when I went off to the British Cycling training camp a month later. The pain went from bad to worse and I was on top of a mountain in Tenerife when I suffered a bout of paralysis. I suddenly couldn't walk. With just nine months to get fit for the Olympics in Rio, it was a disaster. I flew home immediately and had back surgery. At first I found it hard to eat or drink. I couldn't even sit down. But my dream of getting to Rio was big enough. Big enough to get me down to the garage and on the turbo trainer, to make me lie in the back of a taxi just to get to the velodrome and to ride through the pain… You win it when no one is watching.

The why is the motivation insurance. It's what gets you up and out in the morning, come rain or shine, what gets you back on the bike after injuries and illness, what keeps you focused on your riding when distractions and temptations threaten to lead you astray – and they always do. And, it's there for you when it all gets too much and you just want to jack it in. That's why there has to be a reason – the why is the foundation of everything you are doing.

Facts and reality, systems and processes

Professor Steve Peters, the British Cycling team psychiatrist, was a massive part of our success, especially in the 2012 London Olympics. Indeed, I'd say he was as important to the team as Dave Brailsford. Steve's premise was logic over emotion, so much so that Chris Hoy even called him 'the voice of reason'. He taught us the basics of neuroscience, including the role of the limbic system, the part of the brain responsible for our emotional responses. His 'chimp' analogy, which has been central to a number of his bestselling books, compares the limbic system to an inner chimp that acts without our consent or control. The battle is to understand and manage the chimp, which isn't always easy.

When we went out on to the track in an Olympic race, it was a nerve-wracking situation; there were massive expectations and this was potentially a life-changing four minutes. It was a gladiatorial atmosphere and everyone – us, our rivals, the crowd – was buzzing. The adrenaline was pumping, blood flowed to the limbic node and the fight-or-flight instinct kicked it. That's when the chimp can take over. Thinking becomes impulsive, driven by emotion, stress and panic. Plans are thrown out of the window as decisions are made in a state of anger, excitement, desperation and wild opportunism.

It might be an attack on a climb, an attempt to force the pace of the bunch, an escape – they can all be good tactics when considered and carefully judged. Too often, though, they fail because they are rash and, by their nature, ill thought through. Hunger, pain and fatigue all send blood to the limbic system, as does anger. The bunch can be an aggressive arena. Someone is too sharp with their elbows or takes your line and the red mist sets in. if you are not on your guard, the chimp takes over.

Steve Peters taught us to control those moments. The base premise was 'always stick to facts and truths' – don't let emotions get the better of you. He brought everything back to systems and processes. Right from the start, on the beeps, breathing in on nine and out on eight . . . Leaning back for the first 20m . . . into the rhythm and stick to the plan. All you need to think about when things heat up is: what is the situation? How does this support or change my plan? Pragmatically, what is my best option? Take control of your decisions and keep them rational. Concentrate on your own race; shield everything else out. Facts and truths.

> *I was in the 10k scratch race in the Junior World Championship in Moscow in 2003. There were three laps to go and it was looking like it was going to come down to a big bunch sprint. I was a good sprinter; if I floated around the front, I'd have a really good chance of winning. Then in a sudden panic, I made a spur-of-the-moment decision. For some reason I went long. I got away, got a gap and for a few seconds it seemed the gamble might pay off. Then one by one they came flying past me. I finished 26th. Last but one of the bunch.*

It's not about winning or losing: the only race you are in is with yourself.

Motivation and confidence

There's a lot of talk around mental toughness in sport these days. For me, it comes down to two things. First, how much do you like being a cyclist? If you don't love being on the bike, it's mentally taxing to put your heart and soul into it. How are you going to take it to the limit when it comes to doing that last push on the front of the chain gang? Enjoying the sport makes everything so much easier. If you want to be a fair-weather or weekend rider who heads out to the cafe and back, that's great, more power to you. But if your sights are set higher, you'll look forward to every session on the turbo, pedalling through the sleet and feeling the hurt.

Second, how much do you want to achieve your goal? That 'why' can do so much of the heavy lifting when gritted teeth and sheer determination are called for. When you know what your ultimate aim is, motivation and confidence come from following the plan. In the two years leading up to the 2012 Olympics, we didn't plan on a win. What was important was that we showed

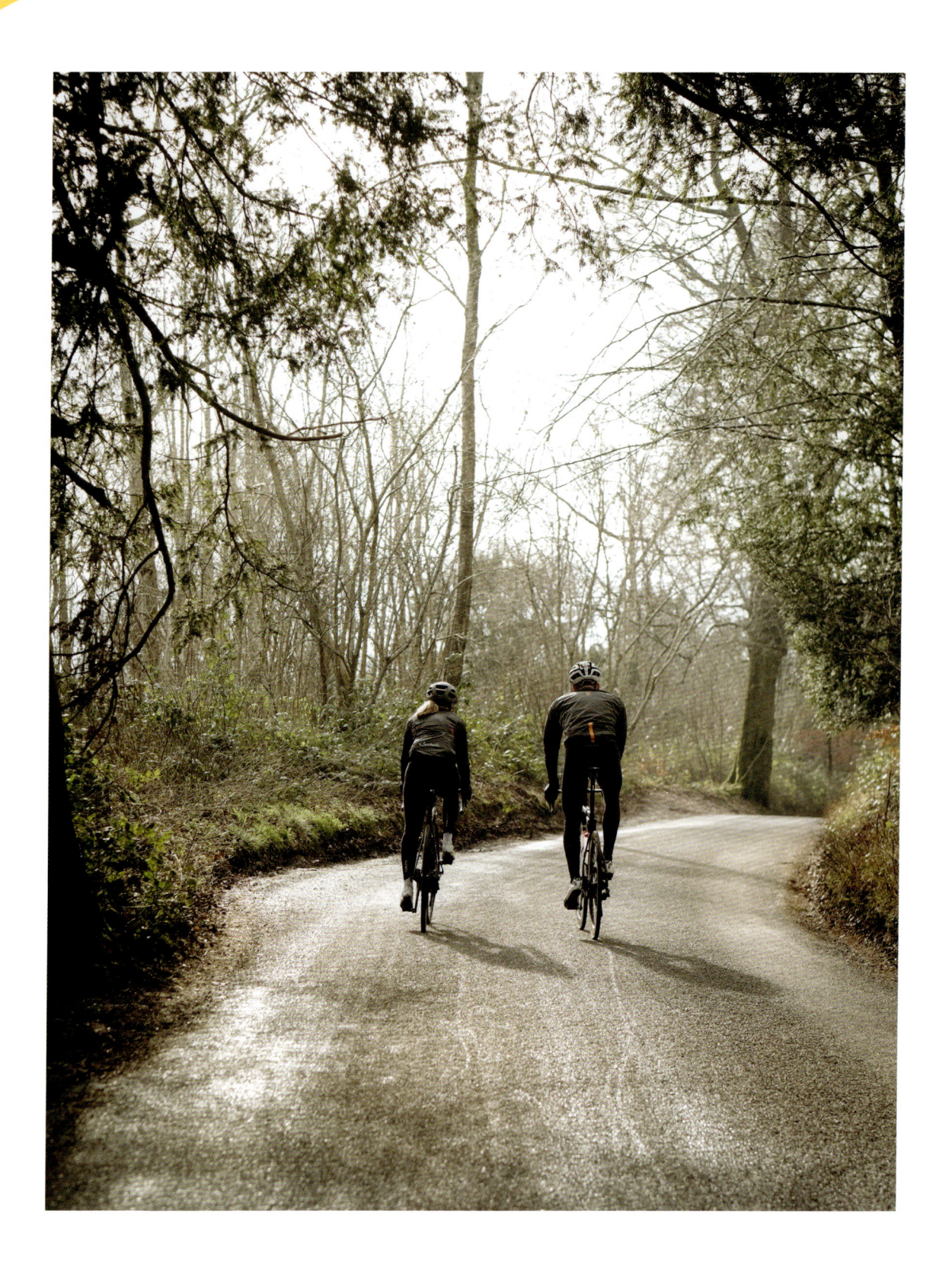

steady improvement. The best have that belief in progression. It's not about winning or losing: the only race you are in is with yourself.

Before big races, at some point I was nearly always asked, 'How confident are you?' After a few stumbling attempts to respond without sounding arrogant or unambitious, I realised there was an honest answer. I got into the habit of saying that I was 100 per cent confident of doing everything in my power, that I had complete confidence in my ability to follow the plan. Control the controllables. I wasn't able to alter the other riders' performances or change the weather, but I could make sure I did everything I was supposed to do.

Feedback

Other people's views are important, but context is always worth bearing in mind. In the GB team we would have analysis immediately after a race. These 'hot debriefs' were taken in the heat of the moment. People – riders and coaches – often spoke without consideration. It was the truth and nakedly honest, but it was coloured by the emotion of the race. 'Cold debriefs' a day or two later gave people time to mull over the race. Observations were more pragmatic and rational. They were broader, with small details forgotten or overlooked. That too was useful, though it could be blunted by sensitivities and politics.

Success

The higher you set your sights, the more you will have to sacrifice. If you are aiming for the very top in sport, it's difficult to be a well-rounded

Mental training

Creating the right mental attitude doesn't happen overnight. As Steve Peters used to say, you don't expect to go to the gym for the first time and walk out ripped and toned. Developing a focused mental attitude takes time, too. You need to become aware of what is happening and what needs to happen in your head. Practise again and again until it's an automatic process and experience it in a real race or a high-pressure situation and see how it stands up. To track how you are progressing and to maintain your focus, try keeping a daily diary noting down:

- What was the purpose of the day? Expect the best results possible.
- Did emotion get the better of intelligence? Reflect on what happened and what could be done.
- List three positives – even if it's just good flat white or the traffic was clear.

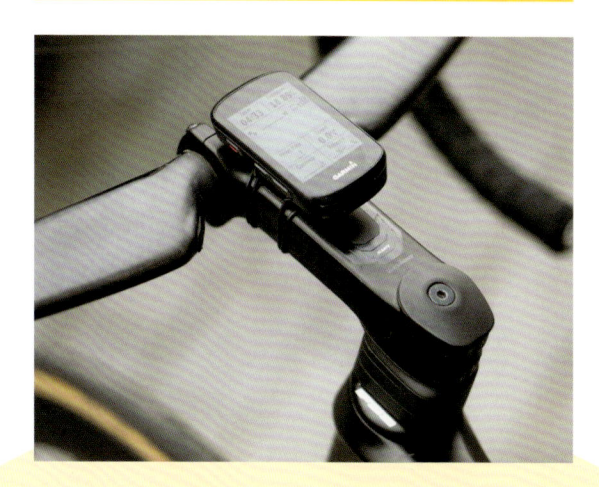

FULL GAS FOREVER

> **Success is not just winning bike races or being the fastest on the sportive. It can just be staying healthy, riding a century or climbing to that mountain top.**

character. You just haven't got the time to be a big socialiser or a dedicated family person. I have heard it said that people become Olympic gold medallists because they aren't any good at anything else! For some, though, midlife is a time when pressures ease up. Work might have become less pressurised, social commitments are less hectic and kids are doing their own thing.

Ultimately, you decide what success is. Success is not just winning bike races or being the fastest on the sportive. It can just be staying healthy, riding a century or climbing to that mountain top. These days, success to me is going out and playing on an electric mountain bike or going full gas on a chain ride.

Setbacks

Nothing goes right forever. Loss of form, an injury, a run of bad luck or an issue unrelated to cycling can derail anyone. Accepting that is the first step. Then you can concentrate of how it fits in with your timeline and what needs to be adjusted to achieve your long-term goal. Perspective is such a useful tool against negativity. Trust the process. Improvement is rarely a linear route. There will almost certainly be backward steps, stagnation and false dawns, but zoom right out and you'll find an upward curve.

Don't exclude yourself or suffer alone. Keep attending events or training sessions. Keeping in touch with teammates and coaches will spur you on to get going again. Make use of your support network, too. The help of family and friends can be invaluable in changing your attitude. People are always kinder to others than they are to themselves.

Give yourself a break. It's unrealistic to think that you can be switched on 100 per cent of the time and it's better to take your foot off the gas now and then than to burn out. Some riders seem to have a phobia of rest days or weeks and that can be far more detrimental that easing

Give yourself a break. It's unrealistic to think that you can be switched on 100 per cent of the time and it's better to take your foot off the gas now and then than to burn out.

up. Rest and relaxation can be an integral part of overall improvement.

So, don't worry if sometimes you just can't face getting on the bike. Even the most motivated athletes have days when they can't be bothered. Build rest days – even allowing for unplanned ones – into your plan. If you find those days stretching to a week and more (I've spent weeks not even getting on a bike), then build a new routine to get you back into the groove.

Regular training can get boring and repetitive. It might help to add some variety; get on the turbo trainer or take a mountain bike off-road. Occasionally on the track, we'd get out the heavy old spoked-wheel bikes just to change things up a little.

Pain

Fausto Coppi famously said, 'Cycling is suffering.' He wasn't wrong, but it's not necessarily as bad as it sounds. When you are out riding or on the turbo trainer nearly every day, your body can get pretty used to the exertion. You can even get to enjoy that dead-behind-the-eyes pain, in a 'it's hurting, so it must be good for me' way.

The feeling of taking things to the limit also holds a certain beauty. I love finding that point where my body is on the edge of shutting down. Knowing that's as hard as I can go and matching my flat out against the others'.

That kind of pain is transitory. You have no control. The only way to handle it is to put it away in a box, knowing it will not last forever. You concentrate on the 'why' and you use the system. Maybe you focus on following a wheel or turning the cranks or getting your teammate to an agreed point. It arrives, you deal with it and eventually it goes. In retrospect, you know it was there, but you have no overriding memories of being in pain.

The sledgehammer pain of an injury is more difficult to deal with, but it's still surprising how much resilience you can build. The toughest people take the knocks and move on. It's like crashing. Many new riders are terrified of crashing, but once you've hit the deck once or twice, you know it's not that bad. Usually you brush yourself down and get back on again.

TRAINING BASICS

Ed Clancy

Training doesn't need to be meticulously scheduled and ultra-scientific. It's just about getting on the bike with a few general guidelines and goals. This chapter covers all the basics, from different types of training to ways to measure output and monitor progression.

It's amazing what can be achieved on a bike, whatever your age. The increasing number of older and veteran cyclists in clubs and rides proves that. However, it doesn't happen overnight. Building up fitness, power, endurance, flexibility and bike handling skills all take time and at least a little dedication. How much training you need depends on your aims, general fitness and the time you have available. You might get by on a couple of hours a week, but if you have a serious goal – sportives, crits, MTB races, étapes – you need to prepare to spend 5–10 hours a week on the bike.

Training doesn't have to be a complicated affair. Even for the elite cyclist, 90 per cent of the training involves spending time on the bike riding at a moderate pace. In Olympic training, endurance riders Bradley Wiggins and Mark Cavendish would basically do the same training as Steven Burke and me, who were short-distance track specialists. The two of us might slope off a little earlier or ease up at the end of the day, but the base was the same. Much is made of thresholds, zones, watts and your VO_2 max – and they can all be helpful in progressing and targeting your performance – but honestly, it can be so much simpler than that. For a start, getting on the bike is only half the story.

50 per cent cycling

We get good at something by doing it repeatedly and cycling is no exception. However, cycling is unique in its merging of (wo)man and machine. Your bike must be fit for purpose and set up for you to perform to your best ability; the same goes for your body. Nutrition and hydration, sleep and rest, flexibility and strength are all key. They go hand in hand with your bike work. You can train like a demon, but without the right lifestyle and preparation, you won't get far – and believe me, I've seen a fair few try. It becomes even more important as the years roll by, when you really do need everything to come together to get it right.

Middle age

The traditional (if not-too accurate) way of calculating your maximum heart rate is 220bpm minus your age. This is one pretty clear sign that age doesn't help fitness. Combined with a steady decline in bone density, muscle mass and metabolic rate in perimenopausal and menopausal women and men over the age of 30, ageing takes its toll and you may wonder whether it's worth the effort persisting with sport. However, the overall effect of ageing on your cycling ability is actually pretty small compared to your lifestyle, diet and training levels. Sure, you may need to visit the gym rather than ride your bike once a week and incorporate some stretching into your daily routine, but enjoying your riding, going faster and further, and even competing, are all still within reach.

Base training

The majority of your time on the bike should be spent cycling at an intensity that feels comfortable rather than forced – zone 2 or 60–70 per cent of your maximum heart rate (*see* p.96). You should be able to conduct a conversation while you ride, but to the point that anyone listening would guess you are exercising. Even five or six hours a week riding at this level is enough to begin to build a training base.

Professionals can spend about 80 per cent of their workout time in zone 2. This is because it is where you train your body to use fat rather than carbohydrates as fuel. Your fat reserves are extensive while carbs are limited, so you are able to ride increasingly faster and longer. It also helps strengthen your heart and blood flow so fewer pumps are needed for effective circulation. The difficulty is holding back and riding slower than you might wish. Your natural inclination will be to push the effort higher, but learn to resist the urge. There's no need to worry: the time to push yourself will come soon enough.

> *The overall effect of ageing on your cycling ability is small compared to your lifestyle, diet and training.*

> **Tip:** take a tiny lock along with you. It takes 30 seconds to nip into a shop for a bottle of water or a banana, but so many cyclists don't stop for fear of their bikes being stolen.

Whatever your cycling discipline, you need the hours on the bike. I rode pursuit, an event that lasts under four minutes, and yet preparing for the event involved 20–25 hours a week on the bike. There was no getting out of it – and believe me I tried. Without the base training I'd soon feel exhausted and after two or three days I'd be on my knees. You soon get burnt-out and feel tired and depressed.

Those hours on the road help in other ways, too. You become comfortable in the saddle for long periods, you get to perfect your bike set-up, and you learn to feed and hydrate correctly, before, during and after a ride. You discover when a sandwich does the job and when a gel is required. Personally, I think hydration advice can sometimes be a little too alarmist. Certainly stay hydrated – don't get to a state where you are thirsty, and make sure you check the colour of your pee (it should be a pale yellow colour) – but you can feel bloated and weighed down if you take on too much liquid.

Training outdoors

Being out on the bike is almost always preferable to sweating it out on an indoor trainer. Sure, it isn't always as convenient, as economic with your time, or as comfortable, but there really is no substitute for the open road. You see the same fitness benefits, as well as developing your bike handling skills and roadcraft, and getting free vitamin D! Choose a country route, or go early in the morning when the roads are quieter, and make sure you are visible. Choose your own time to increase your speed for seconds or minutes. You don't even need a long route, just one decent hill that you can climb then coast back down and attack again at the same or a faster pace. Or find a stretch where you can safely sprint, and then turn around and ride back for the repeat.

Training apps

Free and paid-for apps such as Strava, TrainingPeaks, MapMyRide, Rouvy and others have revolutionised training. They have their own structured training programmes and can be used for route planning and monitoring fitness, and enable you to repeat the same routes and track your times and power numbers over specific segments.

Winter training

The winter months are the season for base training, with plenty of time – at least 10 hours a week – to be spent in the saddle. It can get dull, so many road riders use this time to mix it up with different disciplines such as MTB, cyclo-cross or gravel riding. Also, dark mornings and nights can sometimes limit your ability to spend enough time out on the bike each week. If that is an issue then some indoor sweet-spot training (*see* p. 165) can be incorporated to make sure you are building your fitness.

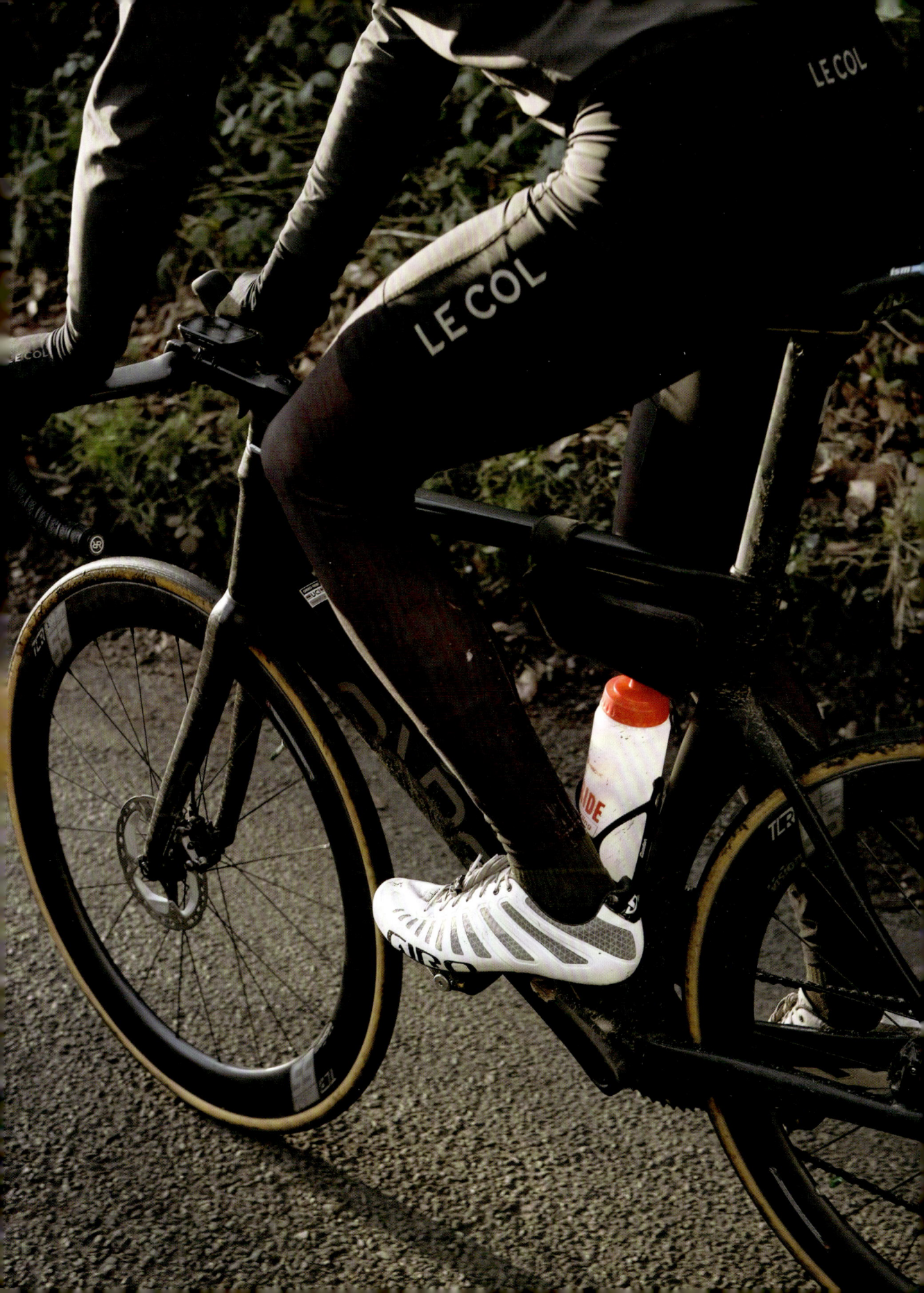

For any training to be effective, be prepared to increase your effort over time. Without pushing your body ever further, your fitness will not improve.

Power meters

Cyclists are luckier than any other endurance athletes in being able to measure their output with a power meter. Heart rate monitors might be a cheaper option and still have their uses, but they are subject to external forces, ranging from nerves to weather conditions to fatigue. Power meters give you a pure and accurate reading of the pressure exerted on the pedals multiplied by the cadence. They have transformed cycling and these days very few riders train without one. They enable you to monitor and optimise your training rides, track your fitness, and help pace yourself through events and races. Used in co-ordination with training apps, they can provide incredible data analysis and there is nothing more motivating then seeing your power data rising.

Using FTP and zones

In many training guides you will hear about functional threshold power (FTP), which is the maximum average power you can sustain for 20 minutes (or an hour). You can calculate your FTP by averaging the power output from some of your toughest 20-minute segments from recent rides or by giving yourself a specific 20-minute test and deducting 5 per cent. It is an arbitrary figure that has no real meaning in itself, but it can be a useful guide to how intensely you train.

However, unless you are riding at elite levels, I don't think there is anything to be gained in over-analysing your output. It is enough to know the general zones you are aiming to train in. At the reasonably easy level you should cycle in during base training (zone 2) you should average around 60–70 per cent of your FTP; tempo training (zones 3–4) is around 80 per cent of your FTP; and anything above 100 per cent (zones 5–7) is all-out full gas. Use FTP as a guide to make sure you are not going too easy or working yourself too hard during different types of training and remember to use it in conjunction with your rate of perceived effort (*see* below).

Rate of perceived effort

Power meters work best alongside a gauge that costs absolutely nothing. Rate of perceived effort (RPE) is a subjective assessment of how physically and mentally tough your exercise feels. Recording your RPE after a training ride will note the external factors that have influenced your performance, such as lack of sleep, hormones, distractions or poor nutrition. Averaging 175 watts an hour can seem easy some days and a real grind on others, and RPE gives some perspective on your performance. It can be on a scale of 1 to 10 (from 1 being very easy to 10 being the maximum) or simpler, such as 'easy', where you can hold a conversation, to 'moderate', where breathing interrupts a sentence, or 'hard', where two or three words are the most you can muster.

Progression

For any training to be effective, be prepared to increase your effort over time. Without pushing your body ever further, your fitness will not improve. Begin low and be prepared to make steady, but gradual, increases in the duration, frequency or intensity of your training. This doesn't mean it has to be more stressful every time you get on the bike – you can increase the stress when you feel ready. You will also need to build in recovery periods.

Carbohydrate-fasted training

This is an increasingly popular method of developing your body's ability to use its fat reserves as fuel, if you are a man. The story is different for women (*see* below). It's not as drastic as it sounds. If you ride first thing in the morning, just have a cup of black coffee and skip breakfast. Your body is used to using carbs as fuel but will be forced to use fat and will become more efficient when called to do so on long rides. However, it comes with a small warning: stick to rides under two hours in duration at an easy (zone 1 or 2) pace and take a gel, banana or flapjack in case you need a boost or want to be conventionally fuelled to continue riding.

The limited research available suggests that fasted training is not advisable for women as the stress on the body can cause hormonal imbalances that can lead to increased fatigue, anxiety and disrupted menstrual cycles.

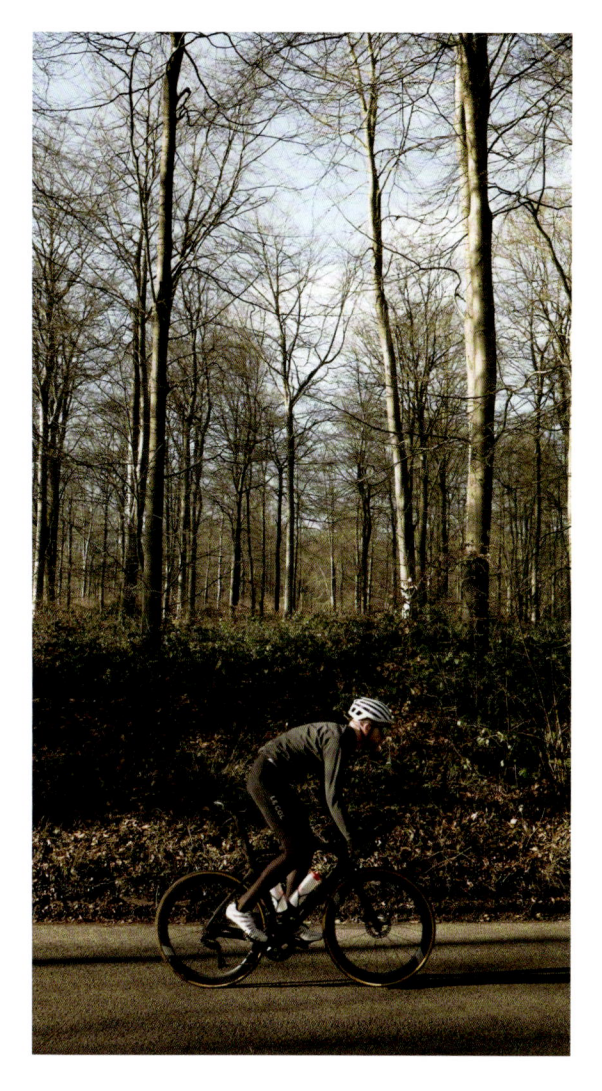

Basic training tips

- Have a routine. Set aside regular times for your training rides, otherwise it is too easy to start skipping sessions.
- Build in your commute. Rides to work or to other engagements all count, so make them part of your plan.
- Be zone-disciplined. Sticking to low-intensity riding can be difficult, but make it a habit.
- Progress. Regularly step up your training, but go long, not deep. Keep the same intensity, but ride for longer or further.
- Don't use not being able to get out on the bike as an excuse. Use an indoor trainer where necessary.
- Include gym sessions, stretching, yoga/Pilates and other sports, such as swimming and running, in your training programme.

Good training is about what you are wrapping it in as well as what's going on with your pedals.

Head for the hills

The difference between a novice and a seasoned rider? One dreads going uphill, while the other welcomes the challenge. It doesn't take long to love the hills; they break up the monotony of long, flat roads and help improve your aerobic capacity and muscular endurance. You don't have to go harder just because it is uphill; you can lower your cadence accordingly. If you are aiming for any event riding or club rides, the chances are you will face anything from one long hill to a day full of climbing. The only real way to prepare is to include them in your training rides. It is not just about the aerobic and anaerobic benefits, but also finding your most comfortable body position. If there's a scarcity of climbs in your area, then find the steepest and longest that you can repeat or circle back to.

Solo or group riding

There are pros and cons in training in groups and training alone. A small group can provide encouragement and motivation as well as enjoyable company. You learn to ride in a chain gang, draft and form echelons, as well as communicating with and overtaking other riders. However, if you have specific training goals or are riding with a group that doesn't push you, it can be frustrating. Solo riding requires focus and self-motivation, but the route, speed and rest stops are entirely down to you. Usually, a mix of the two according to your training goals is the optimum choice.

Training camps

Warm-weather training camps have exploded in popularity over the last decade for all levels of cyclists. Mostly situated in destinations around the Mediterranean, they virtually guarantee warm weather and can provide accommodation and food, challenging cycling routes, back-up, expert advice and massage.

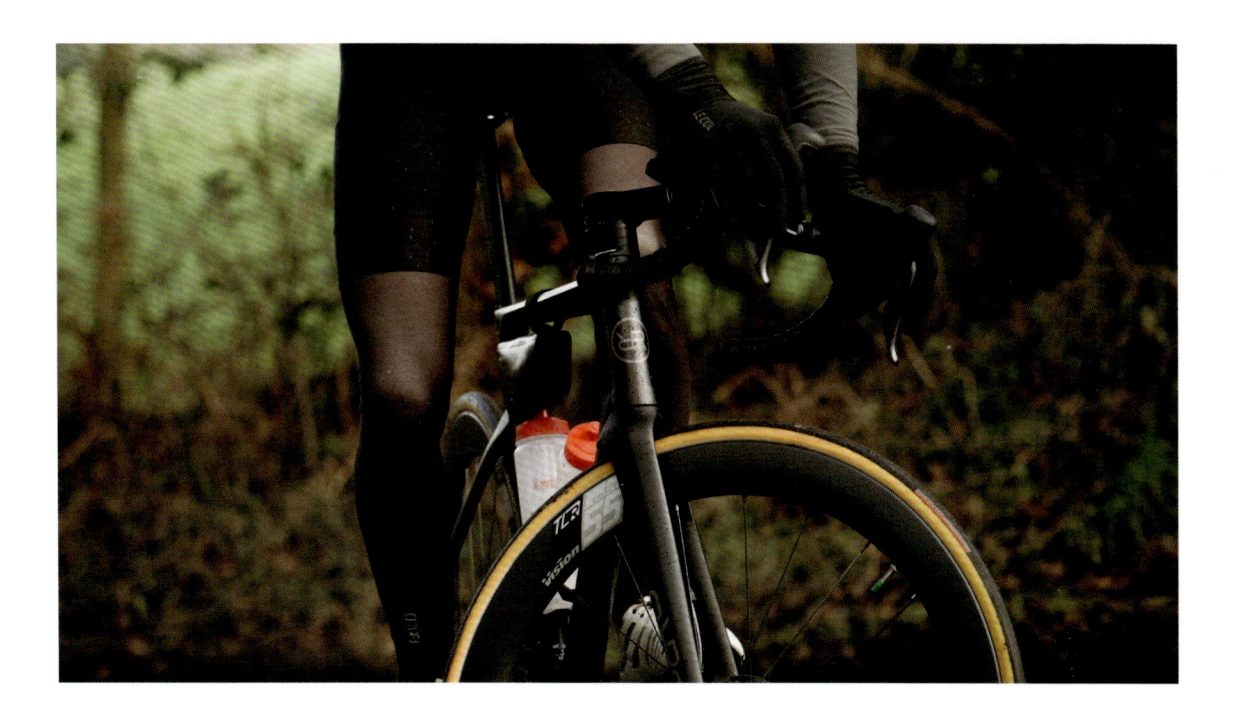

If you've trained through a tough winter then the prospect of a week or two in the sun is pretty mouthwatering. I live in West Yorkshire. It's a lovely place to ride a bike, but the winter weather can be wearing. As soon as I hit the camp in Spain, I can instantly tolerate at least another 30–40 per cent training workload. Home is so full of distractions and diversions, but out there the weather is nice, there's no washing the bike, cooking or other chores; you just ride your bike and rest. Good training is about what you are wrapping it in as well as what's going on with your pedals.

Majorca has become the go-to place, especially the north-east of the island. Recently, it has perhaps become too popular as well as costly and busy, so maybe look for alternatives. Girona, put on the map by Lance Armstrong, is dry, warm and central. It has now gone viral with a huge cycling scene and is a particular favourite of the hipster gravel riders. Personally, I love the Costa Blanca area around Calpe and Altea – it is easy to travel to, and the roads are wide and not too steep. You might even see Tadej Pogačar or Mathieu van der Poel out on the road.

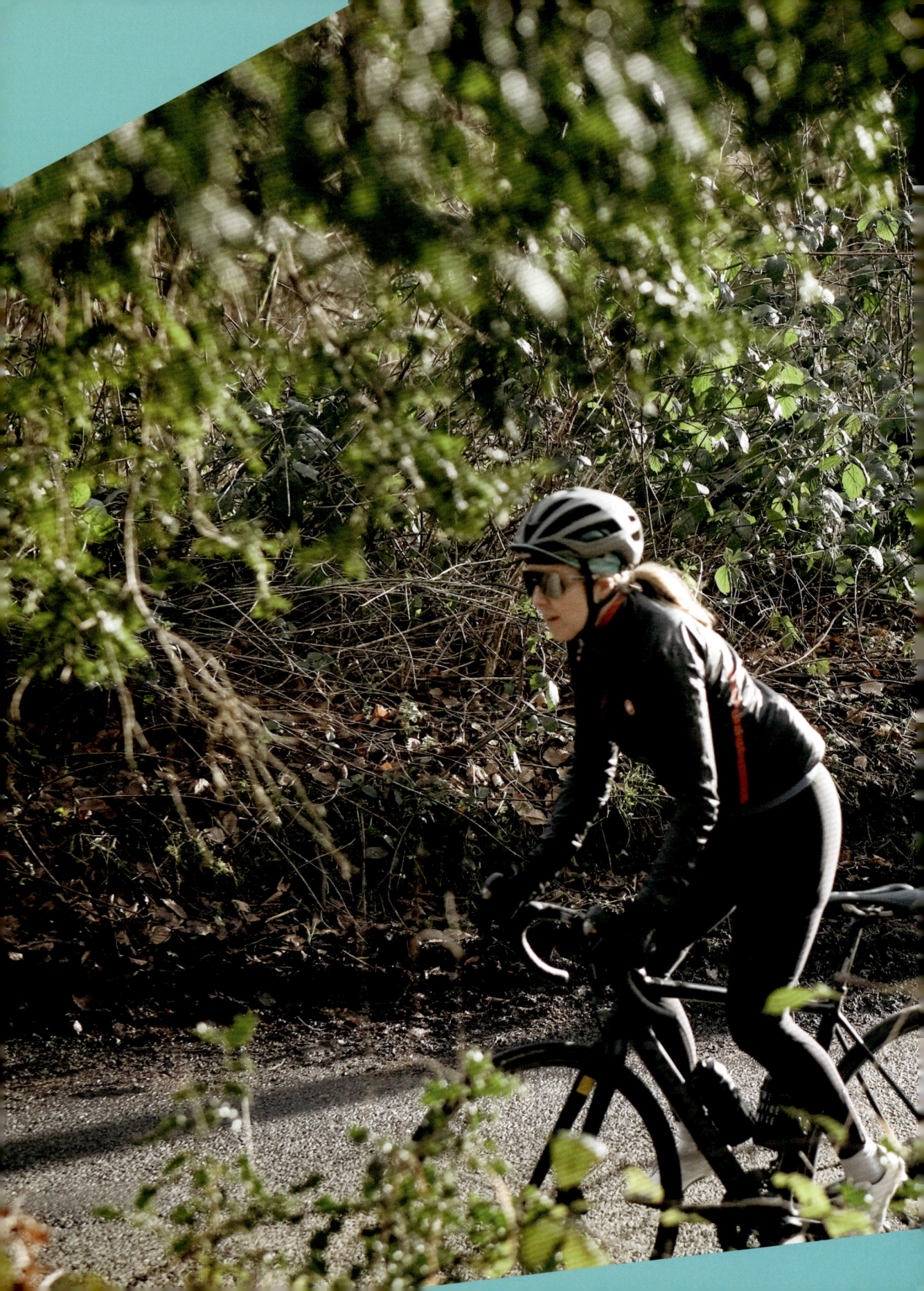

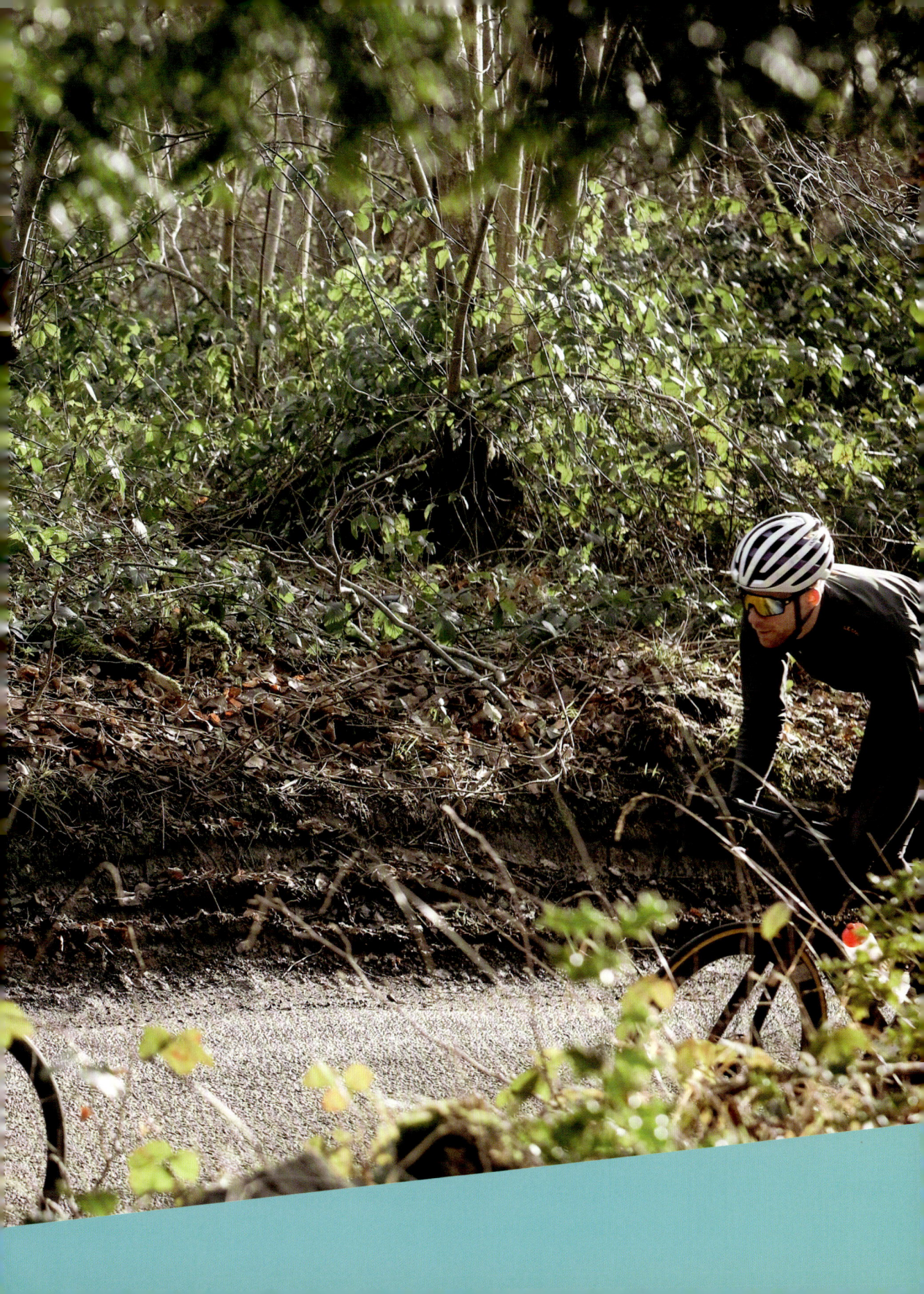

CYCLING TECHNIQUE

10

Ed Clancy

There's so much more to cycling than generating watts. Roadcraft, assured technique and bike handling skills are the foundations of riding faster and are where old minds beat young legs every time.

Fit people aren't necessarily bike riders. I've seen people who look like cyclists get on bikes and really struggle. They can't carry it off for many reasons, but so often it is about technique. Road positioning, riding on someone's wheel, getting in the correct gear, carrying speed round a corner and other reasons to be comfortable, confident and energy efficient on a bike are so important.

As a rider, I've never been too interested in training and physiology. It's necessary and I know I have to do it. I was, however, obsessed with bikes and how to ride them effectively. Bike handling skills, tactical awareness, reading the road – these were the areas that made me a decent rider. I won a lot of criterium races on the road, not through fitness, but because I could ride a bike.

I still remember when my stabilisers came off and my Uncle John let me wobble down the road. I was thinking, 'I'm pedalling and steering and it's all me.' By the time I was in my young teens I was off on my mountain bike all the time, experimenting with saddle height and gears. Then I started racing and an old fella from the Holme Valley Wheelers gave me a pair of clipless pedals and shoes (a couple of sizes too big). It was a game-changer. My pedalling went from stomping on the pedals to a smooth revolution.

Cadence and pedalling

Turning these pedals is, of course, the basis of cycling. It is pretty simple. How fast you pedal in which gear determines how fast you go. Cadence x force = power. Through your gears you can regulate your cadence and maintain a steady rate. That doesn't stop many from trying to complicate matters. You will hear coaches and read manuals recommending 90 revs a minute (rpm) as a suitable cadence for a club-level cyclist, but that really doesn't suit everyone. Cycle at a cadence that feels right for you.

On the track, our bikes were single-speed, one gear. Back in 2004–2005, when I started, it was customary for all the riders in a pursuit team to have the same-size gear – one that everyone could get along with. It was seen as more cohesive. British Cycling broke the mould in 2008 and allowed us to choose our own. I was much happier, even as the guy doing the heavy yards at the start, to have a gear that was 15.25–17.75cm (6–7in) bigger than that of Geraint Thomas or Bradley Wiggins.

We all have fast- and slow-twitch muscles, just in differing proportions. In this context, more fast-twitch muscles are better for heavy work and sprints, while slow-twitch muscles are suited to endurance. I am a fast-twitch cyclist. I push big gears slowly. It is less of a drain on my aerobic system, which was my weaker side. I was strong enough to push a gear, but not good enough aerobically to tolerate a super-fast cadence for four minutes. Geraint wouldn't have had the strength to turn a gear as big as mine for four minutes, whereas I would have exhausted myself before the end mimicking his rate of revolutions.

So try a test, counting for 30 seconds and doubling it to find a cadence sweet spot at which you feel comfortable and can ride fast. Experiment and work out what kind of rider you are. There is no right or wrong. I have a range from 75 to 85rpm – if I try 95rpm, that's inefficient for me, but Ethan Hayter or Geraint produce the same power at 10 revs a minute more than me.

There are, of course, some caveats. Too high a cadence can lead to a lack of balance and can affect your pedalling action. On the other hand, labouring a big gear can cause you to be less reactive and can fatigue you earlier, which could be an issue on very long days in the saddle.

The natural way of rotating the pedals is to push down from just after the highest point with each foot. The advent of

CYCLING TECHNIQUE

Roadcraft, assured technique and bike handling skills are the foundations of riding faster, and are where old minds beat young legs every time.

FULL GAS FOREVER

> **One element of going fast on the bike is having the confidence to be able to slow down or stop safely when necessary.**

clipless shoes has made it tempting to pull on the upstroke, too, to increase the power. It does – but only marginally. Don't pull up forcibly on the upstroke. You are fighting against gravity with muscles that aren't going to produce any meaningful power. It just wastes energy. There is, however, something you can do. Start applying pressure on the downstroke from around 2 or 3 o'clock. Don't pull up on the upstroke, but reduce the resistance by taking the weight off that pedal. It's something you can work on when you're on the turbo and have time to concentrate on your pedal action. Keep practising until it becomes automatic.

Regular changing of the gears is essential to maintaining your chosen cadence. Make sure your bike has a suitable range for all gradients in the terrain you are riding. In Norfolk, you may have a 12–21 rear cassette and never run out of gears, while if I venture out in the hills near me without a 27-teeth sprocket on the back, I will be forced out of a cadence sweet spot within minutes.

Riding out of the saddle is significantly less efficient than sitting, but there are times when it gives you a real advantage. Standing on the pedals generates extra power, as it recruits your upper body muscles and puts your whole bodyweight on the downstroke. For the same reason it saps energy fast and can easily leave you in the red if it's not used sparingly.

On a climb, when losing your aero position has less effect, standing can be particularly useful. You can accelerate much more easily, so often it is used in an attack or to negotiate a short climb or a steep incline. Getting out of the saddle requires a little care. Change into a slightly bigger gear before you get up as you will feel more comfortable at a lower cadence when you are out of the saddle, grip the hoods and push yourself up with your foot at the 12 o'clock position. Lean forward slightly, moving your centre of gravity nearer the front of the bike, and be aware that your body will rock from side to side as you pedal. Don't sway too much, as that is just wasted energy.

The same acceleration can be utilised when sprinting. This time you grip the drops and lean forward with a straight back and your bodyweight over the bottom bracket. Finally, on a long ride, getting out of the saddle briefly will change your riding position completely, and take the stress off overworked and stiff muscles.

Braking

Rule number one of braking: the less you brake on a ride, the better. It is just wasting energy. If you can descend or get round a corner without touching your brakes, then don't brake. Use your head first – looking ahead for corners, riders bunching up or obstacles in the road – and stop pedalling and sit up. If you have to scrub speed, do it lightly with either or both brakes.

That said, every rider should be able to stop quickly. One element of going fast on the bike is having the confidence to be able to slow down or stop safely when necessary. Eight times out of 10, amateur riders will come off before they hit the actual crash point, because they can't stop quickly and effectively. If you just grab your brakes at speed, I guarantee you will fly over the bars. There is a huge weight transfer when you hit the brakes with all the weight on the front wheel.

This is why everything is done on the front brake when you are slowing down quickly. The key is to become an expert at modulating your speed with the front brake. The faster you have to brake, the more you should push your weight back. Stay relaxed, with loose shoulders, bent elbows and a light grip on the bars, which will make it easier to manoeuvre out of trouble.

Cornering

Taking a corner will generally come naturally and doesn't need overthinking, but hitting a tight corner at speed – especially on a descent – can test even the best of riders. Braking harder and later than anyone else will give you a distinct advantage, but it is a skill that needs developing.

First, think ahead. If you can't see the exit from 20m (22 yards) or so away, then it is going to be tight. If it is, as long as the road is closed and it is safe, you will want to make the cornering as wide as you can. Swing wide into it, hit the apex and exit as wide as possible. You are looking for the highest possible minimum speed (when you are at the apex). If the corner is less tight, then make the line as straight as you can.

A novice cyclist will brake far too soon. You don't want to cruise into the corner and you should have plenty of time to approach at speed, with your hands on the drops, giving you a low centre of gravity and good leverage on the brakes. Scrub your speed almost like an emergency stop. Before you turn into the corner, your front braking should be basically finished. Don't go in hot with the front brake. You can't ask two things of your front wheel: it can brake or corner, not both. If you do need to brake on the corner, do it when your line is as straight as possible and favour the back brake at this point; a rear-wheel slide is at least controllable.

As soon as you see the exit from the corner start pedalling again. As you do, lean to the inside of the corner and stand your bike up (moto GP riders do a good exaggerated version of this) to avoid a pedal strike – hitting the inside pedal on

FULL GAS FOREVER

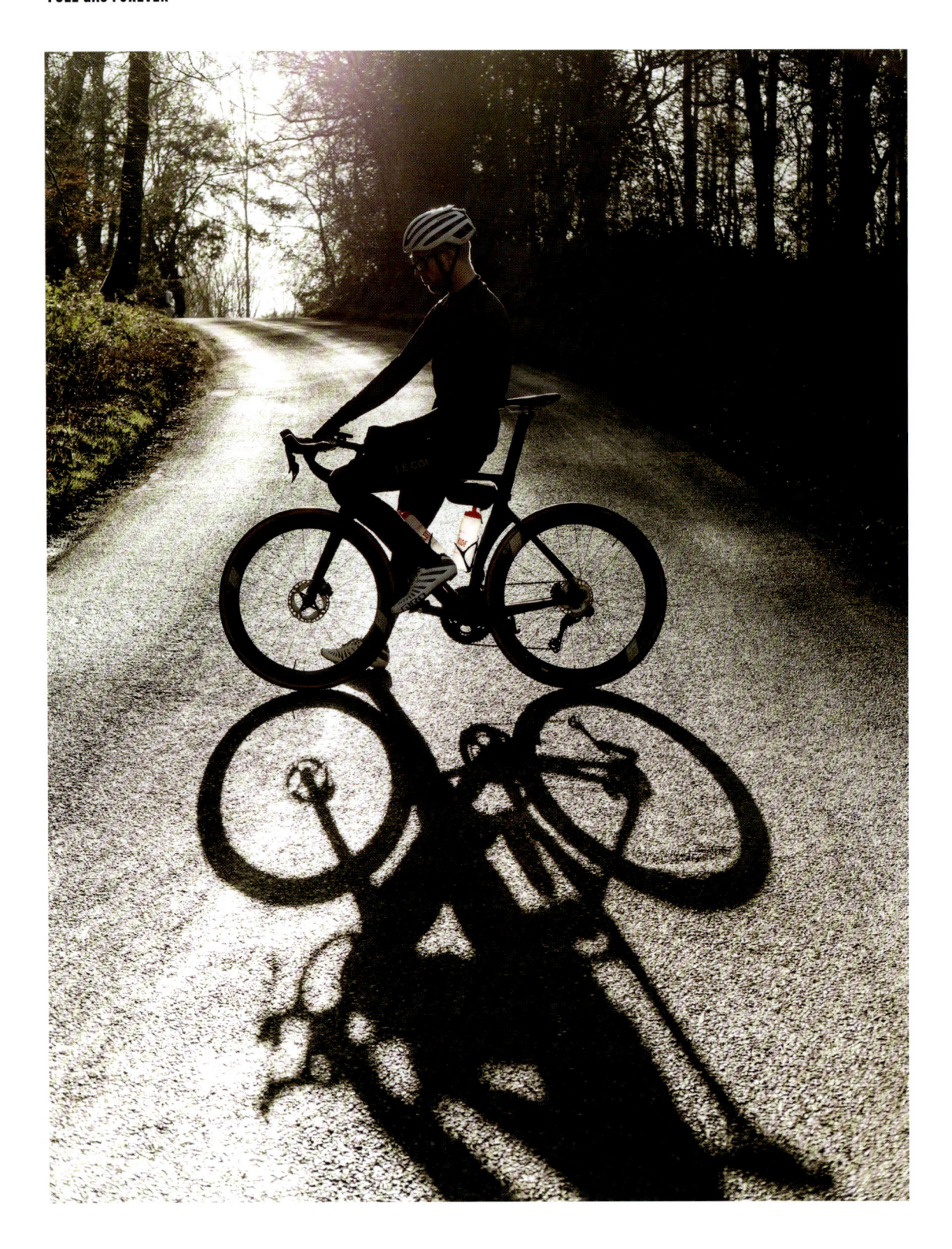

the ground. Flying through a corner is such a great feeling – one of the big highs of cycling.

Drafting

Riding in a slipstream is what makes cycling the best sport in the world and is the basis for so much cycle racing. It makes it possible for riders of varying abilities to ride together and less strong riders to even win races. Obviously it has negligible effect in a tailwind or uphill, but when you have a pan-flat road with a headwind, riding in the middle of a bunch can mean you use as much as half the power as the riders on the front. If you attack on an uphill with a tailwind, then you can be gone, but try it on a bunch with a headwind and you'll be caught in no time.

In order to benefit from drafting you need to be close to the wheel in front, but you don't have to be precariously close to gain some advantage. Whether you are 2.5cm (1in) or 12.5cm (5in) away, it isn't going to make a massive difference, but once you are 15cm (6in) or more behind, the effect drastically drops off. For a lot of cyclists, riding so close seems scary at first, but it doesn't have to be. Sure, you need to be brave, but you can see plenty of the oncoming road and touching wheels doesn't automatically spell disaster. You can let the wheel in front go clear or learn to keep upright when wheels touch. You can practise alone by sitting on the bike and touching your front wheel against a post or ride with others on soft ground, touching wheels and also leaning into each other with your shoulders.

Crosswinds always make for an exciting bike race, as positioning becomes even more important. When the wind comes in at an angle, the optimum place to be is not directly behind the other riders but off-centre behind, so an echelon of riders is formed. You'll feel and hear the correct position.

A crosswind usually hits without warning. Often your response is a simple matter of slightly changing the angle to the rider in front, but the impact of the crosswind can be so dramatic. The only way to prepare is to study a map of the route and the wind direction, and make sure you are near the front at that point. The frontrunners are the riders who realise first and will benefit most. The sooner you get your act together, the better. It works the same in terms of rotating position to share the workload, but the line stretches across the road and there is only a finite amount of space – room enough for 10–20 riders at the most. If you are not in one of the groups and can't force yourself into one, you'll be left in the gutter and will struggle to make any headway.

Communication is key in any bunch riding, but in a crosswind it becomes even more important. The rider in front tends to find it harder to feel where the wind is coming from; it is easier when you are in their shelter. So, the second or even third rider might know better than the lead rider. Let them know where you are positioned and what is happening.

TRAINING SPECIFICS

Ed Clancy

Generating power through the pedal is a high energy-consuming activity. Working on your anaerobic fitness is the answer to conquering the climbs and sustaining the sprints.

Your training through the low-intensity, long-duration rides improves your aerobic fitness – how efficiently your body uses oxygen. Any endurance athlete requires a high degree of aerobic capability. However, you also need anaerobic fitness, especially for the times of fatigue or intensity, when your body can't access sufficient oxygen quickly enough.

It's a simplification to characterise the two systems as endurance versus speed and power, as there is a huge crossover between the use of aerobic and anaerobic energy. Think of it more like a sliding scale, where pootling along is mostly aerobic and full-gas sprinting is almost entirely anaerobic, with much of the pedalling in between relying on both.

Olympic training

My opinion, though others will swear otherwise, and what I've seen with my own eyes, is that there is no formula or breakdown that gives you a golden ticket to success. As long as you are covering the necessary bases, the end result is pretty similar.

Practise for what you intend to do

The first question you should ask yourself is, what am I training for? Are you looking to gain overall fitness, complete a particular sportive, étape, time trial or one-off event, stay with the club rides, ride criteriums, gravel, MTB or other short races, or compete over a season or more? In your training programme, these goals will dictate how much, when and what kind of anaerobic training you do.

If you have put in the right amount of base training over the winter, the pre-season in early spring is when the higher-intensity work begins. It will mean riding fewer long rides and in higher zones but shorter sessions. The aim is to maintain the endurance levels you have built up over the

How and when you work on your anaerobic fitness is down to you. I rode in three Olympics from 2008 in Beijing to London 2012 and Rio in 2016. Before Beijing, I was out on the bike 15–20 hours a week (with half that volume every three or four weeks). We did the speed work early in the season – January to March – then backed it up with interval training, Majorca camp, threshold work and maintaining our strength and power, while also nailing the track specifics such as cadence, starts and team positions.

It was a similar schedule ahead of the London 2012 Olympics, perhaps with more road work, power and strength work on the track, but less time in the gym, and it earned us slightly better results, though we arguably also had a better team.

Then for Rio, we worked with legendary German cycling coach Heiko Salzwedel. We would ride 30 hours a week, sometimes at altitude. They would be long-distance rides with no intensity. Then we would come off the mountain and do nothing but interval training for a week, all power and strength work, then rest. And guess what? That worked too. The training pattern looked so different, but brought the same result.

winter, while increasing power and your ability to ride anaerobically on the bike.

Interval training, which involves working for short periods at a more intense level than your base training, can bring general and specific benefits. Especially useful is that it helps to reduce the natural decline of aerobic capacity as you get older. It can also help develop muscle strength, which enables you to generate more force with each pedal stroke. More specifically, it can improve your climbing, sprinting and other high-effort bursts, such as closing down other riders or escaping a group.

Lactate

When riding at anaerobic levels, the body switches from processing oxygen and glucose for energy to processing glucose without oxygen, producing increasing amounts of lactic acid as a by-product. Your body can deal with a certain amount of lactic acid, but eventually it becomes overwhelmed and the resultant acidity leads to aching and tight muscles. This lactate threshold (LTHR) – the point at which the body cannot clear the amount of lactate produced – is key to performance levels across cycling disciplines. Interval training above the lactate threshold,

There is no formula or breakdown that gives you a golden ticket to success. As long as you are covering the necessary bases, the end result is pretty similar.

while not able to reduce the amount of lactate produced, trains the body to clear the lactate more efficiently and to tolerate it better.

To determine your threshold accurately requires a blood test, but you can find a workable figure with a heart rate monitor. Warm up indoors or outdoors in a low gear and slowly accelerate to your FTP. When your heart rate stops rising and becomes steady, that will be a reasonable figure to use as your LTHR. Be aware that your indoor and outdoor measurements will differ due to your ability to cool down, wind resistance, changes in terrain and other factors. Hormonal fluctuations can also affect aerobic fitness by influencing cardiovascular health, including changes in blood vessel function and lipid metabolism, potentially affecting the efficiency of oxygen transport and utilisation during aerobic activities. You should use the appropriate figure as well as checking periodically for changes. Peri-menopausal and menopausal women should also bear in mind that these measurements can be affected by hormonal fluctuations.

Interval training

With your FTP and LTHR, you have two measurements with which to structure your training. The first thing is to remember that your endurance work needs to continue to maintain the fitness you built up with base training. However, incorporating two 30–60-minute high-intensity sessions a week instead of a long ride should show progress on those key performance indicators.

In order to improve you need to push yourself, but be aware of your own capacity. Work hard when you feel you can and take it easy if you are feeling below par for any reason – we all have bad days and you can do more harm than good. Finally, don't plough straight into high-intensity exercise. Warming up and cooling down should be integral to every training session.

Interval training is the ideal way to improve the energy systems that enable you to ride faster and stronger. By incorporating bursts of high exertion and short periods of rest you are able to extend the time you spend at or above your thresholds. There might be specific formulas suited to your individual aims, but for general fitness on the bike, use a variety – our bodies are adept at getting used to zones and love having new stresses and challenges.

Polarisation and periodisation

Whatever training plan you devise, it will have a mix of intensities. If it has 'polarisation', it will almost totally consist of high-volume work at low intensity and high-intensity work at low volume. Others might choose a more general approach and incorporate moderate-intensity and sweet-spot training into their schedule.

'Periodisation' means changing the intensity ratio as the year progresses in order to reach your goal. The best training plan for you is one that is progressive and interesting enough to stick to. Pro cyclists are training 20–30 hours a week, but your don't need to do anything like that – otherwise it is so easy to lose motivation. Depending on your goals, you can get by with as little as five or six hours – one long ride and two interval training sessions – on the bike each week. If you have the commitment to make sure you do the training you can even be flexible with the times, perhaps fitting in a midweek evening club ride instead of a session.

Overtraining

The amount of workload that you can tolerate and what is 'optimal' will be in a constant state of flux. It is dependent on a range of factors, including sleep, diet, stress, illness, hormones, injury and virtually anything and everything in your life. Pushing yourself is part of the training process, but knowing when to ease up and when to stop is important in preventing injury, illness and disillusionment. Here are some top tips to help you avoid overtraining:

- Use your power meter or heart monitor to keep your training on track.
- Don't overreach even if you feel good. Stick to your training volume. Revise the plan if it is too easy.
- Take note of injuries and rest when necessary.
- Fatigue is part of training, but if you have not recovered after a usual rest then miss a session.
- Progress in small steps, not huge leaps.

Progressing and plateauing

Regular testing of your FTP every month or so should give you an indication of your fitness progress. However, it is not a definitive reading. A number of factors can lead to a fluctuation. You are looking for a steady increase, something around 1–2 per cent a month. If you do not achieve this on any given month then do not retest immediately. Carry on and test again a fortnight later. Do not look for gains above 2 per cent; that kind of increase is simple unsustainable.

At some point it is likely that you will reach a plateau, when progress stalls. Often this is because the body becomes accustomed to the stresses being put upon it. Analyse your training programme and determine if you are not rising to the challenges you have set or you are finding them too easy. Introduce some variation or take an extended rest and return when you have renewed vigour. It may even be that you have just reached your full potential given your work–life balance and commitments. Maybe it is unreasonable to expect to keep improving indefinitely?

Tapering

The idea of easing off your training schedule in the weeks before a race or a big event may seem counterintuitive. Surely you should be trying to reach peak fitness? Nevertheless, most riders will benefit from some kind of rest from the stresses and fatigue of hard training. Tapering involves beginning to reduce the training load – maintaining the intensity but reducing the duration – in the weeks beforehand and having minimal training in the immediate three days before the event. Each person responds differently: some may need only a few days' tapering period, while others will need up to a few weeks. It takes some confidence to believe that you won't lose too much hard-earned fitness over such a short period. Indeed, you might well lose

FULL GAS FOREVER

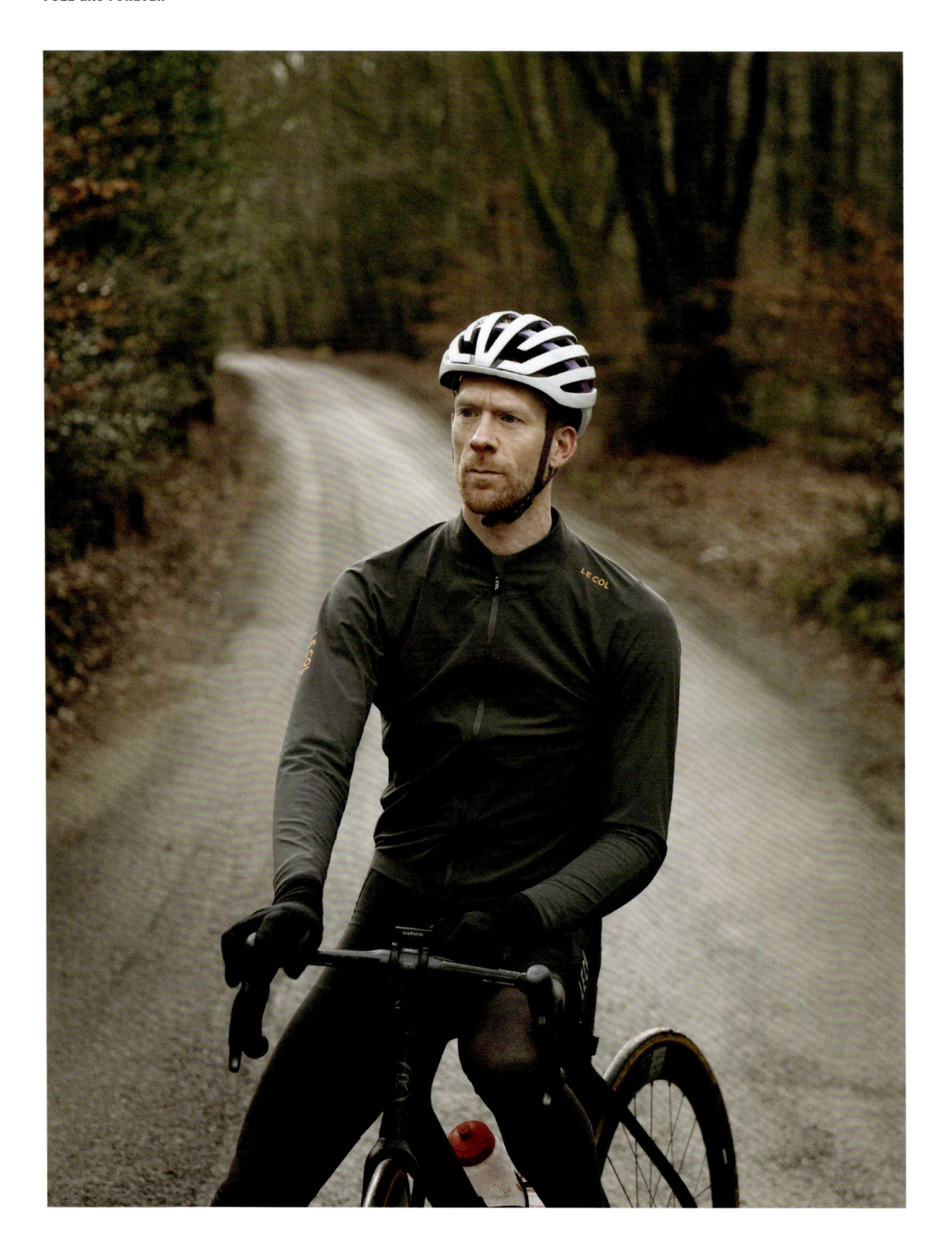

a small amount, but that will be more than compensated for by arriving at the start feeling refreshed.

> Tapering was an established practice when I was racing. It seemed to work well for me, but was less effective for endurance riders like Brad or Geraint. We seemed to get it right for the 2012 Olympics, having a heavy May and June but reducing the effort through July, chipping away at the fluff around the serious efforts. Our numbers in structured training even began to go up and in the final five or six days before the events began, I hardly touched a bike at all.

Devising a training programme

There is no one correct training programme for an event – just one that suits the individual, taking into account their circumstances, lifestyle and other commitments. A training programme that prepares a 25-year-old with no family or other commitments and a part-time job for an étape will be very different to a schedule drawn up for the same event for a 55-year-old man with a high-stress job, a wife and two teenage children, and limited spare time.

Your training programme should reflect the kind of rides you are expecting to participate in. A long, and maybe hilly, sportive that takes up most of the day will need different preparation to an hour-long crit or a club race. They should comprise a mix of endurance work through long rides and high-intensity (indoor or outdoor) sprints and interval training. In theory, do your long ride at the weekend and save shorter, more intense workouts for midweek. Be realistic and flexible, though; life happens and training can always be rearranged. If you miss a session it really isn't the end of the world.

There is no one correct training programme for an event – just one that suits the individual, taking into account their circumstances, lifestyle and other commitments.

EXAMPLE TRAINING PLAN 1

This is an example plan for a stress-heavy and time-poor cyclist with big work and family commitments training for a short club race or criterium.

Sunday

Session: 2.5 hour ride with 4 x 10-second flat sprints

Intensity: Zone 1 on the flat, zone 3 on hills, all-out in the sprints

Instructions: This is your weekly longer ride incorporating flat sprints from a rolling start. Use a moderate gear such as 53 x 17/16 and go zone 3 on the hills

Monday Rest day

Tuesday

Session: 1 hour Zwift/turbo steady ride with 4 x 10-second seated accelerations from a dead start

Intensity: Zone 1/zone 2 throughout with 4 x 10-second seated accelerations

Instructions: This is a steady ride with four accelerations using a big gear from a standing start. Go steady throughout the rest of the ride

Wednesday Rest day

Thursday

Session: 45 minute Zwift/turbo steady ride with 1 x 10-minute block in zone 3 and 1 x 10-minute sweet-spot block

Intensity: Progressive warm-up for 15 minutes, 10 minutes in zone 3, 5-minute rest, 1 x 10-minute sweet-spot block and 5 minutes of cool-down

Instructions: This is a time-efficient light to moderate turbo session working on aerobic power

Friday Rest day

Saturday

Session: 1 hour medium-intensity endurance training

Intensity: Zone 2 on the flat, zone 4 on hills

Instructions: This medium-intensity endurance training will give you a solid tempo session for quality endurance work. Pedal smoothly, stay in an aero position and drink regularly

EXAMPLE TRAINING PLAN 2

An example training plan for a time-poor cyclist to be competitive in a gran fondo or long-distance sportive.

Sunday

Session: 4.5-hour long ride

Intensity: Zone 1 on the flat, zones 2–4 on the climbs

Instructions: This is your weekly long ride – purely for aerobic conditioning (on fatigued legs from Saturday's session). Pace it sensibly in the first two hours and fuel well throughout

Monday Rest day

Tuesday

Session: 1 hour steady ride with 1 x 30-minute block in zone 3

Intensity: Zone 1 for warm-up and cool-down. Middle of zone 3 for the efforts

Instructions: Stay in a good aero position during the effort. Try to find a road that's undisturbed – without traffic light and junctions etc.

Wednesday Rest day

Thursday

Session: 1 hour Zwift/turbo steady ride with 2 x 15-minute sweet-spot blocks

Intensity: Zone 1 on the flat, 2 x 15-minute sweet-spot blocks

Instructions: Warm up for 15 minutes, straight into a 15-minute sweet-spot block, 10 minutes steady, a 15-minute sweet-spot block and 5 minutes of cool-down

Friday Rest day

Saturday

Session: 1.5 hour low-intensity background with sprints

Intensity: Zone 1 background intensity with 4 x flat-out sprints

Instructions: This is a steady background ride but with multiple sprints – 2 x seated on large gear for maximum torque, 2 x from a rolling start out of the saddle at a higher cadence for peak power

HYDRATION

Lexie Williamson

The contents of our bidons gets a lot less airtime than the gels, bars and snacks in our back pockets, but knowing what to drink and how much is crucial to riding performance. Many of us wait to feel thirsty before drinking, but by this point you'll already be seeing a dip in watts and sluggish reaction times. So, let's get some guidance on staying hydrated.

How hydration affects performance

Ever lugged a full bottle or two up and down the hills for hours without drinking a drop because you just kind of forgot? It's super-easy to forget to hydrate, but becoming even a little dehydrated can have significant performance impacts and prolong the recovery process.

There's also research demonstrating that as you get older your body becomes less efficient at producing those 'thirsty' signals and your sweat rate changes, both of which obviously impact us midlife riders.

So, what's happening 'under the bonnet' when we don't take on enough liquid for the ride?

Sweating is a physiological mechanism used by your body to cool down. When you sweat, your plasma volume decreases, which causes a decrease in cardiac output and a rise in body temperature. Your heart struggles to pump blood to work muscles and cool down skin. Result? Your power numbers will plummet and if you've got a lot of tarmac stretching ahead of you, then that's going to feel like an epic struggle.

Deciding to drink at this point won't immediately remedy the situation as it takes time to shunt water from the stomach into the bloodstream. But there are two very simple ways to guard against this. There's the very obvious 'drink enough' (more of which later) on the ride and the not so obvious 'start hydrated' before you pull on the Lycra. But first things first: how much do you actually sweat and, if it's not too personal a question, are you a 'salty sweater'?

Hydrate right in four steps
1) Understand your sweat losses

Sweat rates and the level of dehydration you can tolerate are *highly* individual. Some people only need to glance at the turbo and they've lost litres, while others only barely glow. So, the first step

Research demonstrates that as you get older your body becomes less efficient at producing those 'thirsty' signals and your sweat rate changes.

is to find out how much fluid you lose. There are two types of measurements you can undertake to understand your individual sweat losses: test one tells you how much you sweat and test two says how much sodium you're losing.

I will spare you the details, which can be easily searched online, but essentially for test one you jump on the scales before the session and then again afterwards, and do some calculations to work out the sweat loss.

Test two measures sodium losses. To measure how much sodium you lose per litre of sweat, a 'sweat test' can be completed at rest. Sodium is crucial for water retention. You might already know you're a salty sweater if you can see salt crystals on your bib shorts.

Once you know the results of both of these tests, you will be armed with the data to make decisions over the quantity and contents of your bottles.

2) Drink before you ride

Many of us ride first thing in the morning so are naturally dehydrated. That dark colour of your first pee of the day is confirmation of the eight or nine hours you haven't touched a drop of liquid. Climb straight on to the bike armed with nothing but a swift espresso and you are fighting a losing battle against dehydration.

A couple of cups of water 25 minutes before you get going should be fine for a short or zone 2 ride. If it promises to be a suffer-fest of a session, or is a hot day, it's also worth taking on additional sodium with fluids. Sodium is the main electrolyte lost in sweat. It is involved in the maintenance of fluid balance and blood volume, and is important for nerve transmission, muscle contraction and cognitive function – all of which are pretty handy in cycling. Just drink up to 500ml (17fl oz) of a strong electrolyte mix (1500mg of sodium per litre/34fl oz).

At this point, I must state that the literature promised I wouldn't need to pee having done the 'two cups of water 25 minutes before the ride' thing (female, bib shorts . . . not an easy feat) but sure enough 20 minutes into the ride I was bursting to go and scanning for suitably dense woodland by the road. It was the same again 20 minutes later. So, wonderfully hydrated, yes, but factor in extra pitstops.

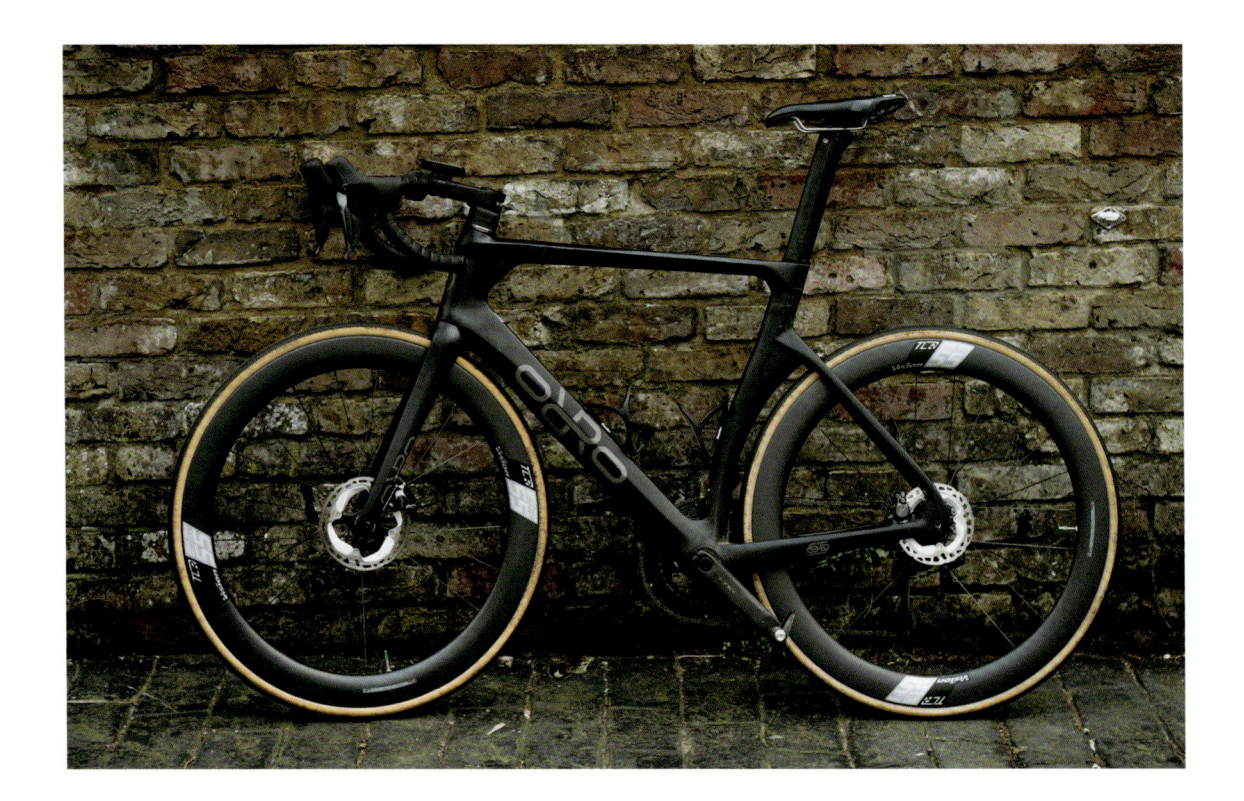

3) Plan what's in your bottles

OK, we've established we need to drink enough, but what goes in those bottles? Electrolyte? Carbs? Or just plain old water? Assuming you're starting the session well hydrated, here's a rough guide to matching your hydration to the session, with help from Emily Arrell, sports scientist at Precision Fuel & Hydration:

45–60 minute turbo

For a zone 2 ride or turbo interval session lasting less than 60 minutes drinking water to thirst is sufficient, unless you are riding or training in the heat, in which case adding a pinch of salt can help with fluid retention. According to Arrell, our bodies can otherwise source sufficient sodium from our usual eating and drinking habits after a short training session.

One to three hour social ride

'For anything over 60 minutes think about incorporating carbohydrates to fuel and electrolytes to replenish those lost in sweat. You can find this combination in the form of an energy drink mix,' says Arrell. Just watch that your body feels OK on the energy drink. Signs of nausea and gastrointestinal issues mean you may have overloaded the gut and not hydrated effectively.

Three hours-plus full-gas ride

'Over three hours and we need to supplement our carb drink mix with gels, chews and bars to

The 'one bottle per hour' myth

OK, it's not really a 'myth' but I got your attention. It's rare to have a chat about hydration without a cyclist confidentially claiming, 'You're supposed to drink a bottle an hour.' But is it true? Emily Arrell says it's not wrong but warns against standardising the amount we drink, as sweat rates vary so highly. A 500ml (17fl oz) bottle an hour might be plenty for some and woefully inadequate for others. If you really want answers, you need to understand your sweat losses first.

meet our basic fuelling needs,' says Arrell. As previously mentioned, you might also be in danger of overloading the gut by drinking a lot of carb mix drink, so it can be beneficial to separate your hydration from your fuel, such as taking one bottle with an electrolyte tablet and another with a carb mix. Then add extra fuel (food) on top.

Big day out in the Alps

Here's where real food comes in. You're just not going to want to stomach another gel after four or five hours in the saddle, so take a break and eat a sandwich. Just avoid anything too fatty or fibrous as the gut will find it tough to digest. At this stage many riders have drunk their carb mix and electrolyte tablet bottles and so switch to plain water but take extra electrolyte tablets with you to pop into these bottles to stop your sodium levels plummeting.

4) Drink enough on the bike

The fourth step is drink regularly on the bike. It's tricky to say exactly how much you should drink as we all sweat at different rates. Some people require a bucket under their indoor trainers while others merely sweat a few drops (see step 1) Understand your sweat losses' on p. 116).

Otherwise, the American College of Sports Medicine suggests about 250ml (8fl oz) every 20 minutes, or just take a couple of long glugs if you don't have a measuring jug in your back pocket.

Does dehydration cause cramp?

Cramping can be a real pain in the backside/calf/feet for some riders while others rarely suffer. For years it was assumed that poor hydration and/or loss of electrolytes through sweating were the primary causes. Recently, though, theories have explored the idea that overstressing muscles and the nervous system by riding hard for longer than you're accustomed to might also be implicated. The current consensus among researchers is that muscle cramps are likely to have multiple overlapping causes including dehydration, electrolyte imbalance and muscular fatigue. So, tailoring training to your racing goals is obviously important but increasing sodium and fluid intake can also still be impactful, especially for those whose cramps come in later in long, hot rides when sweat losses will have been high. In a nutshell: cover all bases because no one knows for sure what causes cramp.

Forgetting to drink?

Regularly arrive home with a full bottle or two and feeling thirsty? It can be difficult to remember to drink during a fast-paced ride, and relying on a feeling of thirst to remind you is not a great idea; even if you don't feel like drinking you could still be dehydrated and, in turn, underperforming. Try setting a timer on your phone at regular 15–20-minute intervals to remind you to take two to three good-sized gulps. Don't wait until you are dry-mouthed and dying for a drink. Very dark yellow pee, and not needing to stop and urinate, are two signs you're not drinking enough.

Coffee Q&A

1. Is it dehydrating?
No. You may have been told that caffeine is a diuretic, which means it causes the kidneys to make more urine, thereby potentially affecting hydration levels on the bike. But it's hard to find science to back this up. The University of Birmingham studied 50 coffee drinkers who consumed between three to six cups a day and found that coffee 'when consumed in moderation by caffeine habituated males contributes to daily fluid requirement and does not pose a detrimental effect to fluid balance.'

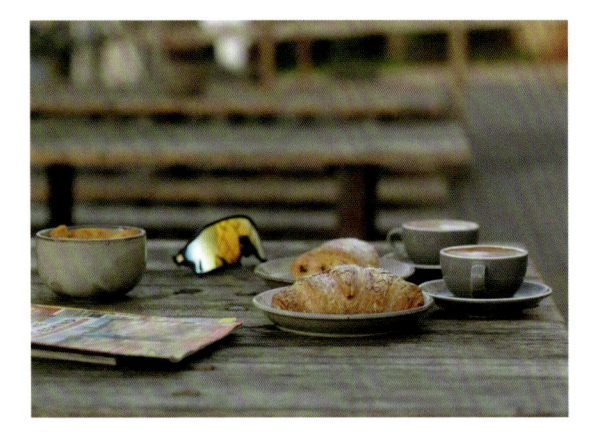

2. Does it help you burn fat?
The jury is out with this one. One study reported a 'highly significant but small' effect of caffeine in increasing fat metabolism. Another suggested you'd need a staggering seven cups if you weigh 68kg (150lb) to have any effect. Since three to four cups is the recommended daily limit, you are probably better just to ride harder.

3. Does it mess with your sleep?
Yes, but you knew that. Caffeine increases the firing of neurons and release of adrenaline, making us feel wide awake. Have that last coffee by 4 p.m. at the very latest if you want a nice, deep slumber.

4. Does it make you faster?
The only question you're really interested in. And the answer is a resounding 'yes'. According to sports physiology, coach and lifelong cyclist Jonathan Baker PhD, caffeine: 'Enhances endurance performance by mobilising fatty acids, thereby sparing muscle glycogen and extending the duration of exertion before fatigue. Secondly, caffeine stimulates the central nervous system, increasing concentration and reducing the perception of effort. It also triggers the release of epinephrine [also known as adrenaline], a hormone that prepares the body for exercise by increasing heart rate, improving blood flow to muscles and elevating the body's ability to metabolise fats. Finally, caffeine may increase the production of endorphins, which can elevate

mood and reduce pain perception during strenuous exercise.' Studies back this up, with one caffeinated group of time triallists improving their times by a startling nine seconds. Boom!

5. How much is too much?
Coffee metabolism is an individual thing. Some folk have the fast metabolising gene and barely feel the effects. Most, though, will get jittery after four cups a day. Beyond this you risk headaches, palpitations, dodgy tummies, anxiety and insomnia.

How to caffeinate a ride
Want to maximise the performance effect of coffee on ride day?

Resist the urge to crawl out of bed and straight to the coffee machine on ride day. Drinking it on an empty stomach can trigger the release of stress hormones like cortisol and adrenaline, which can cause gut issues and begin a spike/crash cycle of energy that continues through the day. Drink water first to rehydrate after sleep, then eat a solid breakfast (oats/yogurt/berries/toast) then go outside (dog walk?) to get some daylight on your skin. Now you are primed for your first coffee. It takes 10 minutes for the caffeine to kick in and 15–20 minutes for it to peak in your system, so drink your first one just before you set off. This one coffee will continue to enhance performance for up to four hours so, according to science, you don't need another one unless you are going on a seriously long spin, but a second one halfway through a three- or four-hour ride will do no harm and also means you can eat that large piece of carrot cake.

Recovery shake

Here's a recipe for a recovery shake you can make at home.

2 heaped scoops of protein powder of your choice or a large dollop of full fat Greek yogurt

350ml (¾ pint) milk (preferably whole cow's milk, which contains fat-soluble vitamins and extra calories)

2–3 frozen bananas (to add thickness and provide carbs)

handful of fresh or frozen blueberries (for vitamins, minerals and fibre)

optional pinch of salt (if you had a hot, depleting session)

optional spices, such as cinnamon (for flavour)

Do I need a recovery drink?
Not if you are meticulous about hydrating and ensuring you consume both carbs and protein after your ride, but why not just tick all three boxes and sip a recovery shake as you stretch (OK, perhaps I'm asking too much here). It will replenish your glycogen stores and fuel muscle synthesis as your body switches from that active, fuel-burning 'catabolic' state to the 'anabolic' or rebuilding stage. It will also tide you over until you can prepare something to eat. No one likes a hangry, sweaty cyclist.

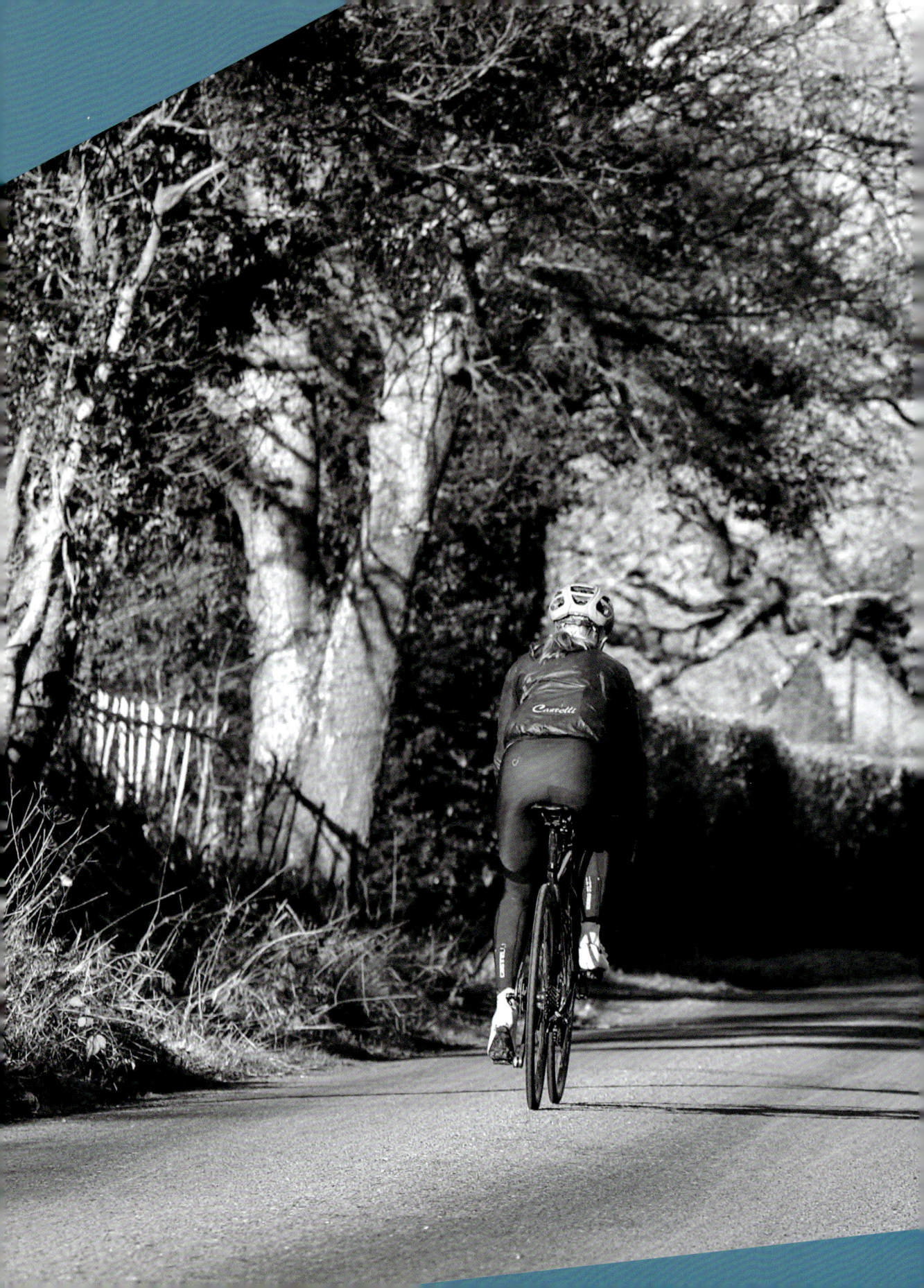

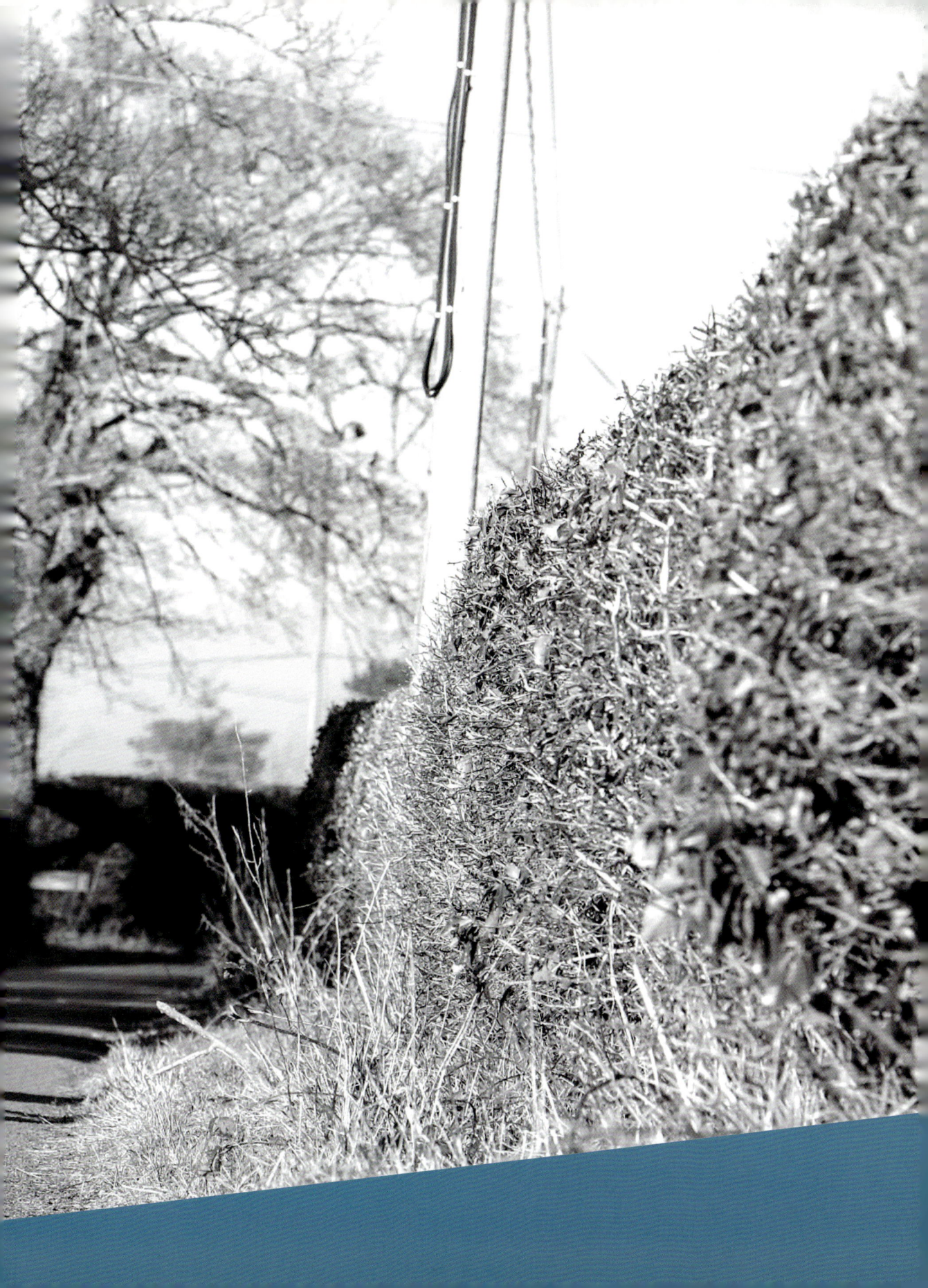

NUTRITION

Lexie Williamson

OK, hands up who has arrived home after a long ride with a back pocket full of untouched bars and gels, and wolfed down everything in sight? Yep! We all know nutrition is crucial, not just for mid-ride fuelling but also repairing muscle afterwards, but its easily neglected amid the buzz of the ride. Let's find out what the Masters cyclist should be eating, with a little help from our experts.

Nutrition and the older rider

So, how should we adjust our nutrition to better suit our requirements as Masters athletes (love that title). As our muscle mass reduces (sarcopenia), our metabolic rate slows, making it harder for us to keep the weight off. The way we metabolise food and store energy as carbohydrate and fat also alters as we become less insulin-sensitive, according to Phil Cavell in his book *The Midlife Cyclist*. Midlife athletes also need more protein than younger ones due to anabolic resistance, or a declining ability to use the amino acids from proteins to synthesise muscle. The amount of protein recommended for the more mature rider per meal is surprising (*see* 'Protein, protein, protein' on p. 126) although the exact amount required is still debated. Female midlife riders also have weight gain due to the perimenopause and menopause to contend with, as well as fatigue through insomnia that leads many to reach for the chocolate bar over those home-made, low-sugar berry, oat and flaxseed bars (who has the energy to make them if you've been awake since 3 a.m.?). They may also need to take iron and calcium supplements.

This is really getting depressing and it doesn't need to be. A healthy diet (which you probably already have as a keen amateur rider), in addition to some strength training to maintain muscle mass, is an amazing start to countering all of the age-related issues above. Let's see what else we can learn from nutritionists who work with the pros about supplements, gels and knowing your leucine from your creatine.

As our muscle mass reduces (sarcopenia), our metabolic rate slows, making it harder for us to keep the weight off.

How to fuel for the ride

In his book *The Cycling Chef*, Michelin-starred chef and sports nutritionist Alan Murchison gives us a good idea of what to eat first on a rest or light training day and then what to add for hard training or race day. The light day basics are breakfast for slow-release carbs in the form of oats or a piece of toast, perhaps with an egg for protein. Lunch could be pasta, rice or a bagel with chicken, and dinner might be vegetables with meat, fish or pulses. Keep snacks to nuts and dried fruit, avoiding sugary biscuits and sweets. For tougher training days or race days factor in slow-releasing complex carbs such as wholegrain pasta or brown rice two to three hours before any long session. 'Snack like a pro' on the bike for any ride longer than an hour, as longer rides burn glycogen (muscle fuel). For this, Murchison recommends making your own bite-sized snacks (try his book *The Cycling Chef on the Go*, for recipes). Then, 30 minutes before a ride, top up with faster-releasing carbs such as a banana. Post-ride he recommends a home-made smoothie to rehydrate and take in carbs, protein and electrolytes.

To gel, or not to gel . . .

. . . that is the question. Murchison is not a big fan, except in emergencies. The 'texture, taste and sensation' of real food is simply more appealing and the body is accustomed to digesting it, and absorbing and distributing nutrients. 'It isn't, however, accustomed to a number of irregularly ingested liquid shots that bypass much of the system and provide massive boosts of energy,' he explains. The primary aim of mid-ride food is to provide fuel – aka easily digestible carbs – so vitamins, protein, fibre or fat are surplus to requirements. His suggestions include rice cakes, bananas, dates ('so good you'd think they were designed for cycling') and dried fruit.

FULL GAS FOREVER

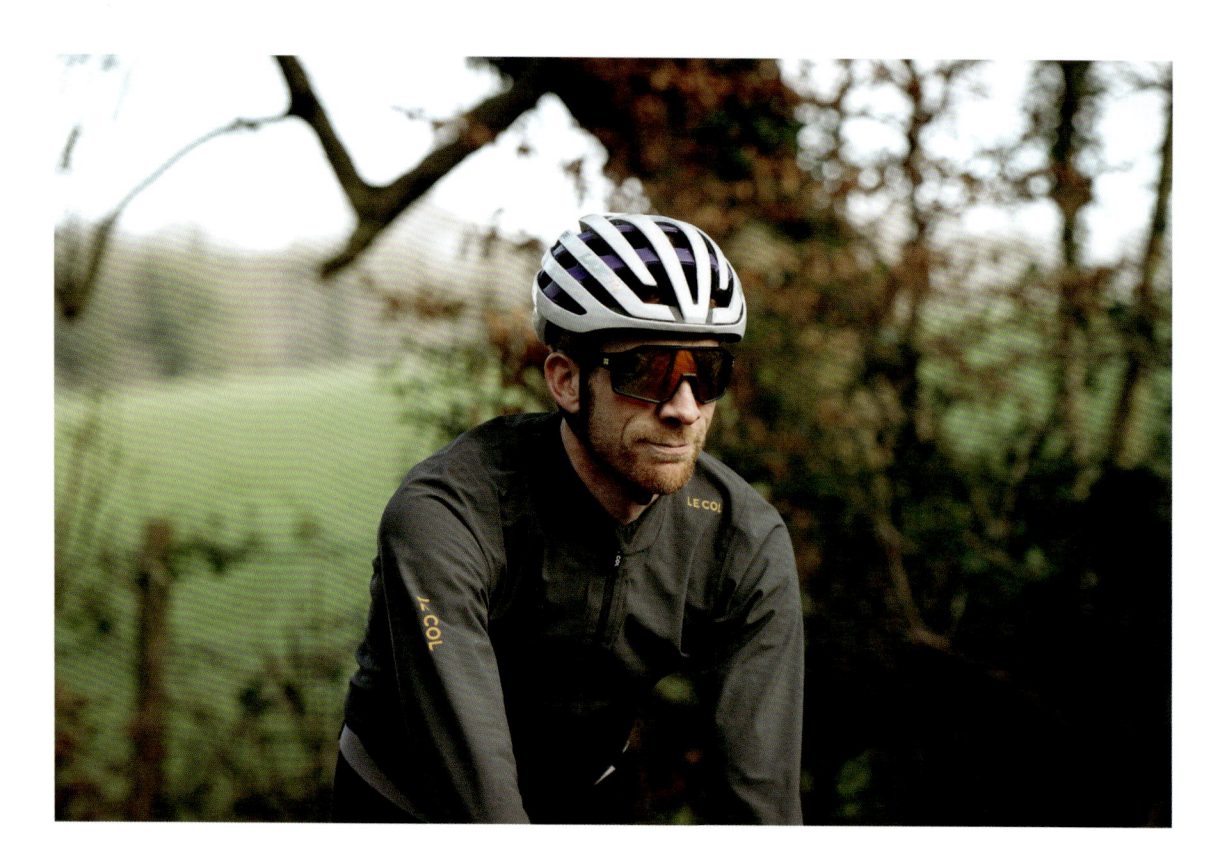

Protein, protein, protein

Did I say protein? If there's a theme that pops up a lot in discussions over nutrition and older cyclists, it is the need for us to consume more protein than we did when we were youngsters. Why? First the bad news: as we age, our muscle naturally degrades, resulting in a drop in performance. This is called sarcopenia and a big cause of it is 'anabolic resistance', which is the declining ability to cause the animo acids from protein to synthesis muscle. In *The Midlife Cyclist*, Phil Cavell says that younger athletes looked after by British Cycling typically consume 0.3g of protein per 1kg of bodyweight every three to four hours. Middle aged or older riders should increase this; aim for at least 30-40g protein per meal. That equates to five eggs or four cups of milk, which is probably far more protein to pile on your plate than you might have guessed! According to Anita Bean, author of *The Complete Guide to Sports Nutrition*, creatine comes out top for the Masters athlete (that's you, by the way), especially when combined with strength training. Protein from meat tends to contain more leucine, which is an essential amino acid that acts as a precursor for protein synthesis and muscle growth. This makes it an important protein for older riders fighting against age-related muscle loss. But leucine also exists in cheese, eggs and fish, as well as quinoa, nuts, peas and soy beans.

Super supplements for the midlife rider

Walk into any health food shop or chemist and there's a baffling array of vitamins and minerals. Many are not necessary, but the supplements below remain steadfast essentials when fads for others have come and gone.

1) Vitamin D
Vitamin D is crucial in protein synthesis and helps us absorb calcium, but as you get older the skin's capacity to produce it from UV light diminishes. Add in factors such as lack of UV in the winter (and the British 'summer') and the fact that most training plans include at least one indoor interval session done under a lightbulb rather than the sun, and it's safe to say that us midlife riders are probably deficient and need a supplement.

2) Omega-3 fatty acids
Unless you eat a lot of oily fish it can be challenging to get sufficient omega-3 fatty acids, which has anti-inflammatory benefits and is thought to help with protein synthesis, from your daily diet. Buy a high-quality supplement rather than cheaper cod liver oil. You can also boost your omega-3 intake by eating flaxseeds, pumpkin seeds, walnuts and chia seeds.

3) Calcium
Because cycling isn't weight-bearing, if we become obsessed with it to the exclusion of other sports (sound familiar?) such as running, it can make us susceptible to osteoporosis and osteopenia. Osteopenia is the loss of bone mass or bone mineral density which, without treatment, can lead to osteoporosis. Bone density starts to decline from age 30. Phil Cavell has met many ultra-fit clients who report back to him with a borderline, or osteoporotic, DEXA score. (A DEXA scan is a type of X-ray that measures bone density.) If we don't eat enough calcium the body will take it from bone stores. It's possible to get enough calcium from food. Options include sardines, milk, yogurt, green leafy vegetables and broccoli, but if you are vegan you might consider taking a supplement or consuming calcium-fortified plant milk.

4) Iron
This is not so straightforward. An iron deficit can make you feel exhausted and frustrated with your poor performance. However, it can be toxic in high quantities and may affect the absorption of other minerals that the body requires. If you are unsure, get a blood test done and speak to your doctor.

FULL GAS FOREVER

Don't skip carbs in a bid to lose that stubborn midlife belly fat. The greater your bodyweight (muscle mass) andexercise volume, the more carbs you need.

The myth of the 30-minute 'recovery window'

OK, calling it a 'myth' is not entirely accurate, but let's just say that the commonly held view that you have a window of 30–45 minutes to gulp down that post-ride protein shake or else that window slams shut is a little overblown. Yes, that shake will stimulate muscle protein synthesis and helps your body repair muscle damage if consumed immediately after a session. Some studies have also found it beneficial to combine protein and carbohydrate in this immediate post-ride snack. But it is also thought now that the 'anabolic effect' (the state where the body builds and repairs muscle tissue) of exercise can last for 24 hours or longer. So, the post-ride protein fix is undoubtedly going to help you hit those daily protein intake goals, but you need to keep topping up on protein throughout the rest of the day and possibly into the next. It is best to distribute protein intake throughout the day rather than consuming it in just one or two meals, Here are Anita Bean's suggestions for post-exercise snacks:

- 500ml (17fl oz) milk/milkshake
- Strained plain Greek yogurt, banana and nuts
- Avocado and egg on toast
- Handful of nuts and dried fruit
- Wholemeal sandwich with tuna, chicken, egg, cheese or hummus

Don't skimp on the carbs

Your ability to store carbs as glycogen in the liver remains as good as you get older as it used to be (at last some good news), so don't skip carbs in a bid to lose that stubborn midlife belly fat. According to Bean, restricting carbohydrate reduces 'exercise economy' (the volume of oxygen the body requires to move at a given speed) when training at moderate and high intensities (64–90 per cent VO_2 max) and reduces performance for high-intensity endurance rides. In terms of carb intake, just keep it simple: the greater your bodyweight (muscle mass) and exercise volume, the more carbs you need. For exercise lasting longer than an hour, consume 30–60g (1–2oz) of carbohydrate per hour. That might be a banana or a gel.

Nutritional pitfalls for cyclists

- **Under-fuelling on rest days** – Eating less to lose weight on rest days will leave you feeling flat and empty on the following hard training day due to lower glycogen (stored form of glucose).
- **Crash dieting** – Training on an extreme calorie-restricted diet might promise rapid weight loss, but can lead to muscle loss, bone density loss and nutritional deficiencies. If you need to lose weight, go for slow, steady and sustainable weight loss that won't affect your training.
- **Under-fuelling on the ride** – This leads to you coming home ravenous and overeating (usually the wrong food). If you fuelled correctly, you shouldn't feel starving afterwards.
- **Trying trendy diets** – These can include diets that are high-fat, low-fat, carnivore and perhaps even vegan (unless carefully monitored and supplemented). Eat all types of food to ensure you get all the fats, carbs, protein and nutrients required for the demanding endurance sport of

Alan Murchison's 'eating rules'

Eating can be a confusing business. Here are some nice, clear rules from Alan Murchison's *The Cycling Chef*:

1. Eat real food – the body processes nutrients from whole food, be it meat, fish, fruit, veg or grains, most effectively.
2. Eat optimally – match the training load with appropriate fuelling.
3. Eat protein – 1.5–2g of protein per 1kg of bodyweight every day to aid recovery.
4. Opt for simple water and plenty of it to hydrate.
5. Watch the fat content of cheese – parmesan is a lower-calorie option.
6. Be snack smart – try home-made energy bars, muffins, nuts and berries.
7. Beer and wine are calories without nutrients, so go easy.
8. Pick natural sugars found in fruit, honey or maple syrup over refined sugar.

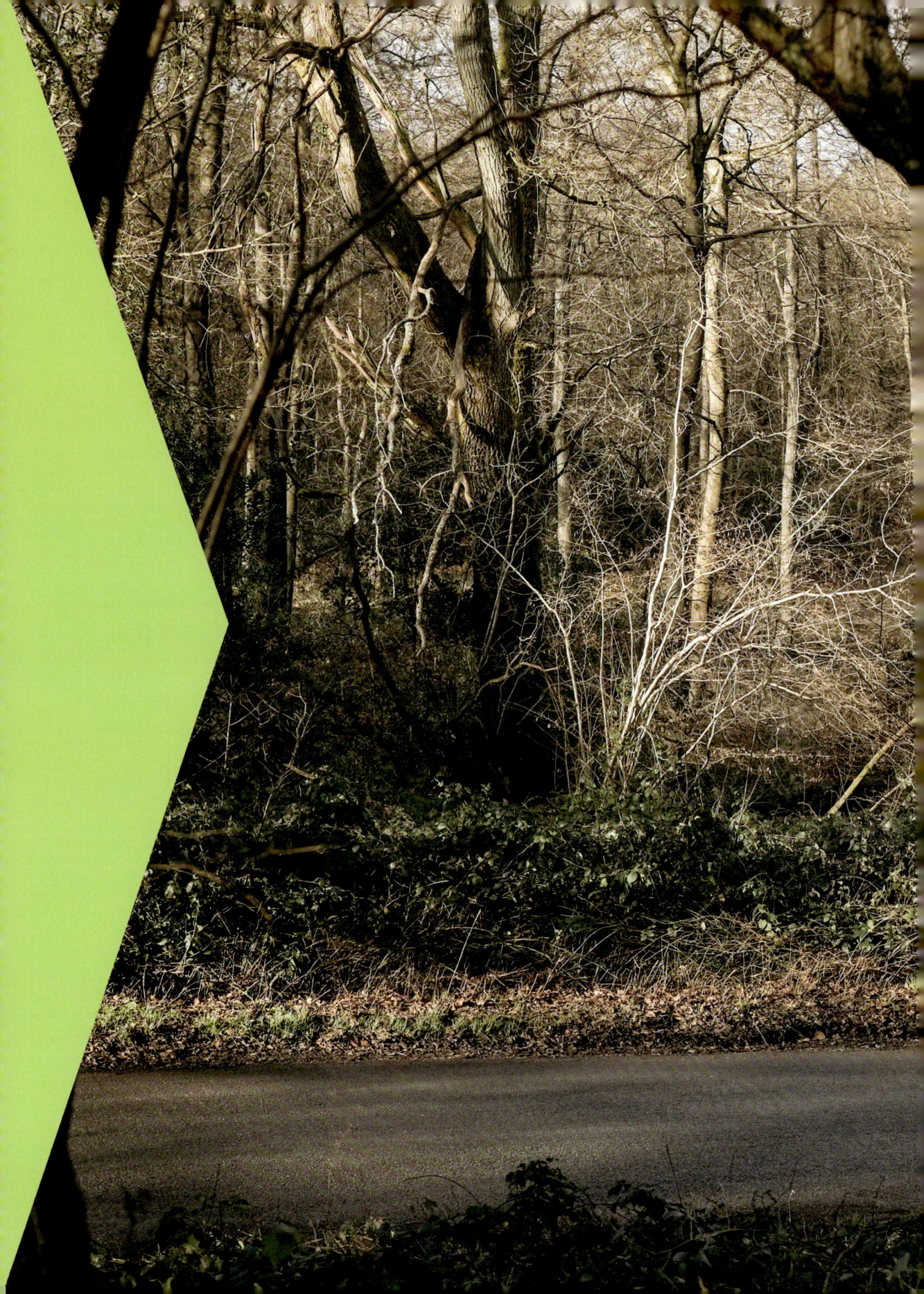

NUTRITION

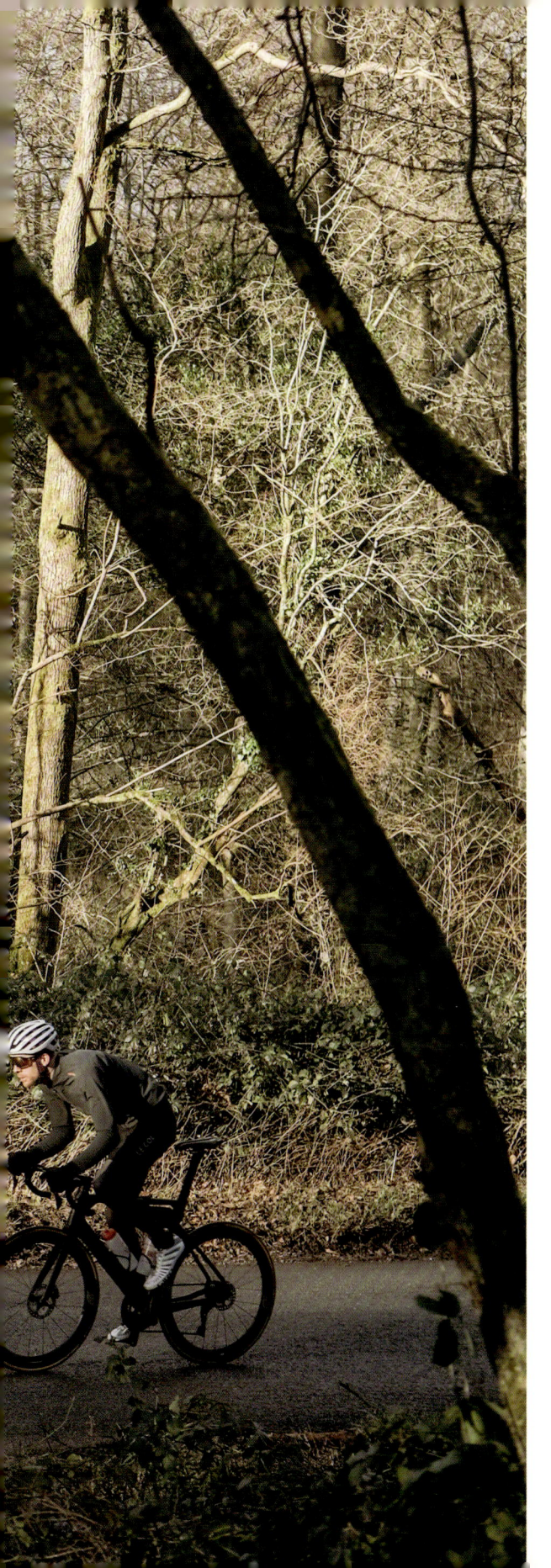

cycling. It's just not the time to skimp on the essentials. If you are vegetarian or vegan, you need to pay close attention to what is required and you may need to take supplements. It is best to consult your doctor or a dietician for advice.

If you have any specific dietary requirements or medical conditions, such as diabetes, intolerances, allergies or GI issues, please speak to your doctor or dietician about your specific requirements.

The pre-bed protein fix

All those hours you spend sleeping are a great opportunity for some sneaky protein synthesis. According to Anita Bean, 300ml (10fl oz) of hot chocolate (or hot milk) contains 10g (⅓oz) of protein, but to up your intake add 20g (⅔oz) of casein protein powder. Or opt for 250g (1 cup) of full-fat Greek yogurt (the authentic stuff, not the 'Greek-style yogurt') mixed with berries and granola, which provides 20g (⅔oz) of protein. Yes, yes, you'll need to get up to pee after all that hot chocolate, but just think of your muscles and all the extra watts they'll produce.

All those hours you spend sleeping are a great opportunity for some sneaky protein synthesis.

131

RECOVERY

Lexie Williamson

If you've bought this book, then my guess is that you're keen to continue to push hard as the years roll by. But should you rest more as you age? There's no doubt that forging on regardless without adequate recovery can mess with your metabolism and hormones, and actually impede fitness improvements, so it turns out that getting older might mean more days off.

Older cyclists' rest requirements

As older cyclists we know we need to factor in more rest; everyone tells us so. But who wants to lose the precious fitness we worked so hard to achieve? Especially as it takes more blood, sweat and tears to achieve it now than it did in our 20s. So, what do we really know about recovery and ageing? It is thought that recovery appears to take longer after 35–40 years of age. Roughly speaking, riders in their 20s and 30s can soak up three or four hard training days and two or three easier days a week. For cyclists in their 50s the hard days drop to two or three, with three or four easier days. Those aged 60 and beyond should probably train hard one to two days a week, although they can still do four or five sessions spinning out the legs.

It sounds pretty conclusive that along with the mounting years comes the need for more rest days, right? But here's the big caveat: recovery, just like training, is *highly individual.* You might be able to push as hard as you ever did, in which case the general consensus on ageing and recovery just may not apply to you.

There is also a bit of a void when it comes to research into age-related differences in recovery from exercise, perhaps because we are the first main generation to really push cycling into midlife and beyond. Sports science just hasn't quite caught up.

Here are some other things to consider about recovery:

1) It might be in your genes

The kind of muscle fibres you inherit can also have an effect on your rate of recovery. We all have differing proportions of slow-twitch and fast-twitch muscle fibres. Fast-twitch fibres generate high power in a short amount of time, but are easily fatigued (think track sprinters) whereas slow-twitch fibres are more fatigue-resistant. One study found that athletes with a greater proportion of fast-twitch fibres seem to take as much as 15 times longer to recover from the same efforts as those with predominantly slow-twitch muscles. No, you probably have no idea what proportion you have in those quads, but it sounds like the perfect excuse to wheel out when you're struggling to keep up at the next club ride.

2) Refuelling is key

Age is only one factor to be considered in recovery. Post-ride fuelling has to be right. Most of us know to whip up a protein fix of some kind within 30 minutes of training and then maybe chow down something carb-laden like a bagel a bit later on, but that's as sophisticated as some people's knowledge of fuelling for recovery gets. There's a good chance that you might not be consuming enough protein or carbs. Building and maintaining muscle mass becomes more difficult as we age. A shake containing whey protein is a quick, easy fix post-ride. However, your body can only absorb a limited amount of protein in one go (about 30g/1oz), so in order to maintain precious muscle mass, us midlifers need to eat protein throughout the day. Eggs, authentic full-fat Greek yogurt, salmon, sardines, poultry, quinoa and nuts are all good sources. And don't forget that bedtime glass of milk. Midlife cyclists worry sometimes that eating close to bedtime may lead them to put on weight but all those hours you spend sleeping are a neglected opportunity for protein synthesis. Learn from the pros and grab a protein-rich snack before you hit the hay.

3) Sleep matters

Are you clocking 8–10 hours of sleep a night (as well as a 'Nana nap' – *see* p. 141)? Most of us scrape by with less

Riders in their 20s can soak up three or four hard training days a week. For cyclists in their 50s this drops to two or three.

Don't normalise constant exhaustion!

In a nutshell, overtraining is the result of an imbalance between training and recovery. The term 'overtraining' is confusing but we're not talking about bonking on a ride or that general post-ride fatigue that leads to an involuntary Sunday afternoon sofa nap. It's not even that two-day feeling of fatigue after a week-long training camp. Instead, it's the many weeks of exceeding your physiological limits leading to weeks or months of diminished performance.

Here are some clues you might be overtraining:

- Out-of-character feelings of anger or depression
- A resting heart rate that is 10bpm above its normal range (see 'Follow your heart' on p. 136)
- Experiencing lethargy/fatigue on a daily basis
- Suffering with minor ailments such as sore throat or stomach upset
- Sleep cycle disruption, such as waking up in the night
- Getting slower, even after a few days of rest
- A higher-than-normal heart rate variability (HRV) (see 'Follow your heart' on p. 136)

than this, but sleep is crucial to recovery and athletes (yep, that's us!) need more than ordinary mortals to repair muscles, restore hormone balance and more. The advice is to sleep between 8–10 hours a night and as a bonus, top it up with a 20–90-minute daytime nap as this stabilises cortisol levels, which rise during hard sessions, and increases mental acuity (you can relay that to whoever catches you napping).

Now, hands up who gets that much sleep? It's not easy with work stress, family commitments and more to just drop off, and the menopause often gifts midlife female riders with the joy of insomnia. But it's worth having a crack at getting more sleep, as this is when your muscles repair and adapt, and the body releases human growth hormone (HGH), which increases and preserves muscle mass, but declines as we age. For tips on how to get a good night's sleep, turn to chapter 15.

4) It might just be in your head

We're not saying you're lying about your sore quads but there is one study that took place over three days and consisted of 30-minute time trails that studied the perception of fatigue in 'veteran' athletes compared to the youngsters. As expected, the older riders reported more muscle fatigue than the younger cyclists as the days wore on, but, importantly, they showed no corresponding decline in physical performance. They *said* they felt more tired, but their power meters told a different story to their RPE (rate of perceived exertion). So, are we suggesting that the DOMS that you feel in your quads two

Regular structured training (as opposed to overtraining) will help you recover faster whatever your age.

days after that club ride with the fast group is imaginary? No: while the muscles of the older riders performed well in the study, they *perceived* or felt their muscles were more fatigued than the younger group. So, perhaps this relates to the brains or nervous systems of these veteran riders rather than the muscles? This is not an invitation to overtrain, but the takeaway from this is that you might feel fatigued, but your body can still smash that session. Or as Jens Voigt famously put it: 'Shut up, legs'.

Having considered the above, are you still feeling exhausted? Let's look into fatigue and overtraining to see if you recognise any of the signs and symptoms.

The four types of fatigue

These are the four classified types of fatigue associated with athletic endeavours, according to the sports science world. Professor Samuele Marcora, specialises in the effects of physiology and psychology on fatigue and human performance.

1. Acute fatigue – The normal tiredness experienced by most people after having done a bout of vigorous exercise.
2. Functional overreaching – Higher levels of fatigue over one to three weeks of overload. Performance decreases temporarily, but after deloading, you get stronger. It's an intense but planned block of hard training.
3. Non-functional overreaching – This occurs with sustained overloading. Not enough rest results in burnout, which can take a month to come back from.
4. Overtraining or chronic fatigue – A state of burnout from which the body and brain can take months to recover. The cause is sustained psychological and physical stress over a prolonged period.

Credit: *Cycling Weekly*

Is recovery trainable?

This is an interesting one. Essentially, 'yes' is the answer. Your rate of recovery is trainable. You can improve how well you bounce back from the stress of cycling sessions. Your body can increase its tolerance to this stress and become better at recovering from it, as you become fitter. This is called the repeated bout effect.

Workouts put you in a state of stress, but repeat these workouts and your body adjusts. So, the lesson here is: don't skip sessions (unless you are ill or injured)! In other words, consistency, consistency, consistency is the key to effective training. Regular, structured training (as opposed to overtraining by squeezing more sessions in) will help you recover faster whatever your age.

Follow your heart: RHR and HRV

Resting heart rate
Of course, we have an inbuilt device that can tell us more about recovery (and lack of it) than any app or podcast: our own hearts. Most smart watches and other 'wearables' like rings and wrist bands will give you your resting heart rate (RHR) and heart rate variability (HRV) score or number. RHR is a good indicator of recovery and knowing it will give you a good baseline to work from if you think you might be overcooking the training or getting ill. Measure it at the same time every day using your watch or by hand before you get out of bed and before the teenager/boss/incontinent dog has had a chance to get your heart rate soaring. Using a watch is probably a more reliable way to take the measurement than placing your middle and index finger on the underside of your wrist.

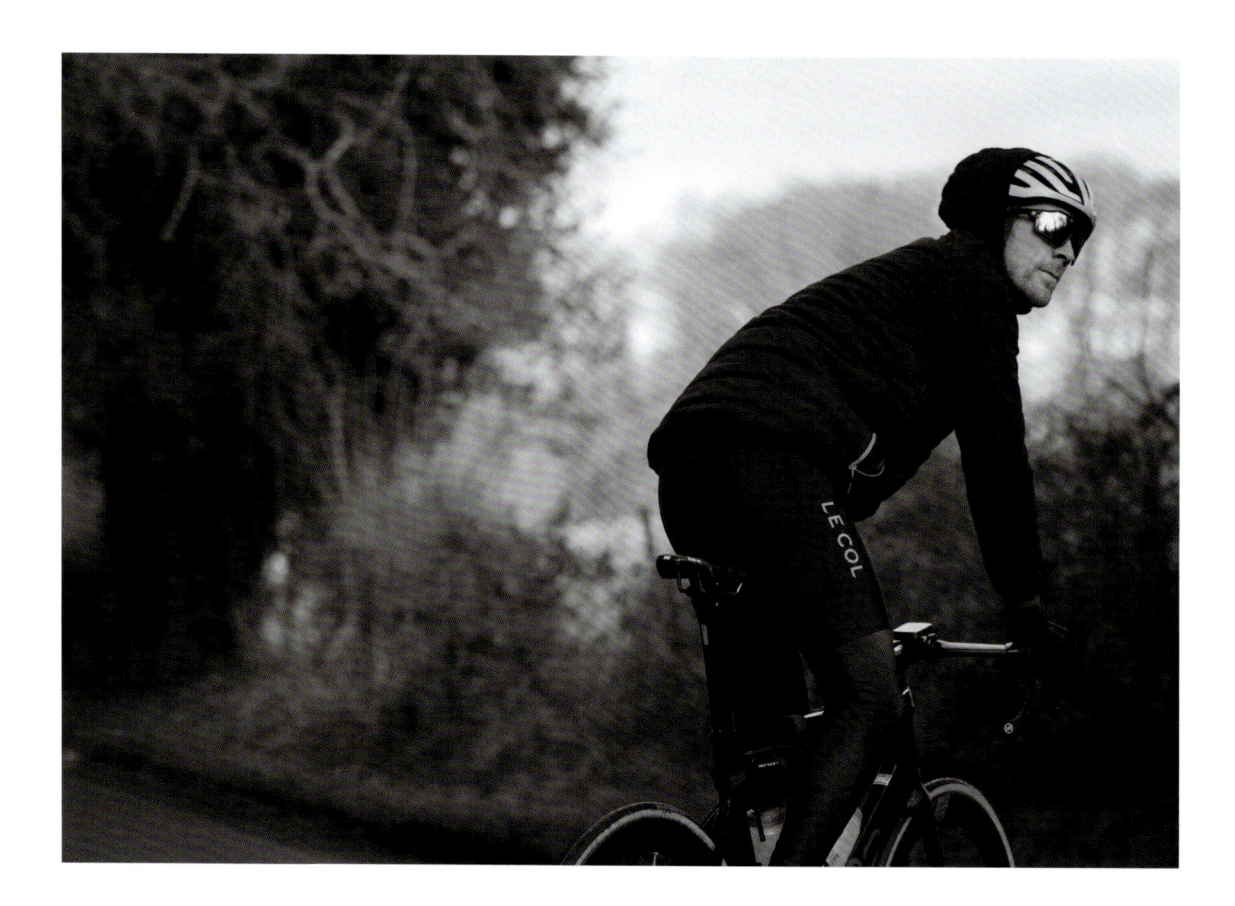

Do this for a few weeks (a month would be ideal) to get a good idea of your baseline number, as your RHR will fluctuate a bit, and take into account any hard sessions, dehydration from drinking alcohol, hard training or hormone cycles. A RHR that is 10bpm higher than normal for several days in a row might indicate more rest is needed or that your body is combatting sickness or is in a phase of the menstrual cycle or hormonal fluctuation that means your body is working harder than normal. Remember also that a gradual decrease in RHR over time with regular training is a good thing!

Heart rate variability

HRV is the variation in time between heartbeats. Rather than having a metronome-like regular heartbeat, it's healthy to have variance, or difference, in gaps between the beats. This is because it may be a sign that the two elements of your autonomic nervous system – the rest-and-digest and the fight-or-flight modes – are balanced. A high HRV number is seen as good and this tends to rise after a good sleep and regular relaxing practices like meditation, which can reduce stress. It can also lower after an intense period of training and could be a sign of overtraining as we stray too far into fight-or-flight (sympathetic) nervous system mode, especially if it continues to be low even if you add in more rest days.

However, there are questions about the accuracy, reliability and usefulness of tracking HRV and more research is needed. So don't stress if you are fit, not overtraining and are not under too much life stress, but still have a low score. HRV also naturally lowers as you age.

Active recovery, aka 'embarrassingly slow riding'

Have you ever done an active recovery session? Yes? Thought so. Technically, you *can* still ride and it counts as 'rest', *if* you take it easy, but most cyclists get overexcited when the endorphins kick in and overexert themselves. Active recovery has to be super slow! Neal Henderson, founder of APEX Coaching and elite cycling and triathlon coach, says of active recovery rides: 'You should feel embarrassed to be seen riding so easy.' Doing it properly will increase blood flow into tired muscles, decrease inflammation and get nutrients to those sore muscles. 'The faster they can repair themselves,' says Henderson, 'the sooner you can stress the body again.' So, if your bike is calling, go to it – and then ride slowly. Just maybe do it at 5 a.m. when you can't be spotted . . .

SLEEP

Lexie Williamson

You snooze, you lose, right? Not according to the pro riders. Cycling teams are taking quality of sleep increasingly seriously due to its proven performance-boosting benefits. So, what hacks for a solid night's slumber can us part-time amateurs pick up from the pros and their sleep advisors?

The importance of sleep

First up, let's find out how sleep (or lack of) can affect your performance on the bike. The biggie here is human growth hormone (HGH). This helps you build muscle and burn fat and stimulates tissue growth thereby allowing you to recover faster. HGH is released as you sleep, the majority secreted between 11 p.m. and 1 a.m. HGH production slows with age, so it's particularly crucial for older riders to go to bed at a decent hour to grab as much HGH as possible.

Sleep also allows us to restock stores of our glycogen (glucose that is stored in the muscles). Glycogen is a big source of energy for endurance athletes, providing fuel when you're working hard, and will be utilised on any ride longer than about 90 minutes. We all know how it feels to deplete these stores and 'bonk' (readers outside the UK might find quite a different definition of 'bonking' if they consult the *Oxford English Dictionary*, but essentially it is slang for that feeling of utter weakness that requires a Coke, immediately).

Sleep deprivation also slows reaction times, which has obvious implications for making split-second decisions on the road or trails, and creates an overactive amygdala – the fear centre of the brain – making us a bit jittery and overemotional. Our perception of suffering also increases and as much as we love to suffer, a good sleep is an easy way to push harder for longer without feeling every pedal stroke.

If you're a bit of an insomniac, this is probably not helping, as the last thing you need is added pressure to get your eight hours a night. But there are a few nuggets of good news for those who can find sleep challenging due to age, a headful of work/family stuff or the delights of the menopause.

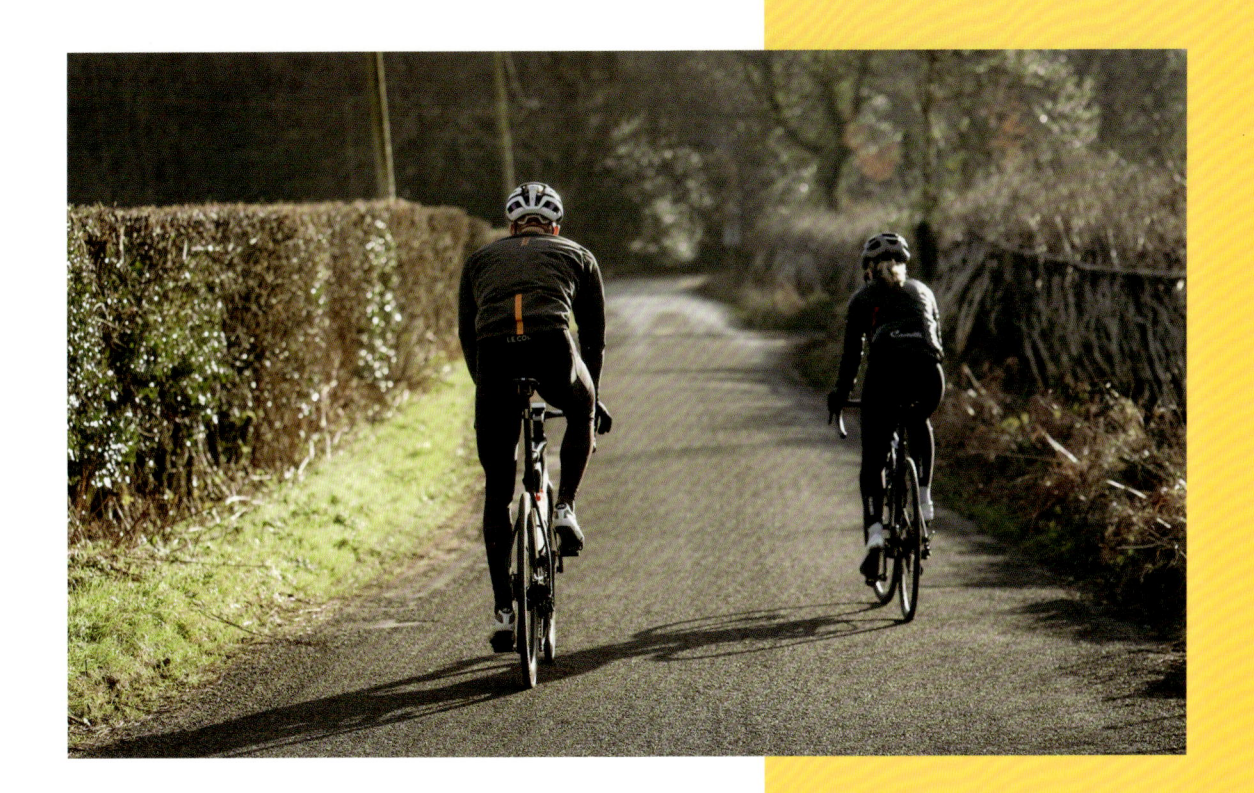

The first upside is that studies have found that one sleepless night doesn't negatively impact endurance or power. This means you might toss and turn before a big ride or race and your performance won't suffer, so don't sweat over the odd night spent staring at the ceiling here and there.

You can also top up your nocturnal sleep by having a bit of a lie-in. There has been research on the performance benefits of 'sleep extension'. A study found that cyclists who extended their sleep time by 90 minutes for three days improved endurance performance by 3 per cent in a 60-minute time trial. So go to bed earlier or sleep in a bit later to secure this top-up.

And the best piece of news is that napping is officially a training and recovery tool; a fact to share with the family as you enjoy some horizontal time on the sofa after that taxing Sunday morning ride and are being asked to cook the lunch or walk the dog or mow the lawn.

Napping is officially a training and recovery tool.

Sleep hacks for cyclists

So, what can the sleep advisors to the pros teach us about increasing our chances of dropping off (and staying there). Here are a few tips:

- **Eat your porridge in the garden** – Getting some direct natural light when you first wake up stimulates the release of hormones such as serotonin. Our circadian rhythm is attuned to the light–dark cycle so soak up lots of light first thing, less in the evening and zero during the night.
- **Nap for 20–30 minutes** – If you're training hard, but struggling to sleep more than seven hours at night (the minimum amount for athletes), supplement nocturnal sleeping with a daytime nap (see 'Napping: aka 'the siesta for speed' on p. 141).
- **Mix it up** – Aim for seven to nine hours of sleep a night but if this proves tricky, set aside an hour for 'recovery' in the day. Recovery might include a nap, a simple breathing exercise or even just putting your feet up for 10 minutes. Don't get hung up on achieving a set number of hours for your main nocturnal sleep.
- **Don't train too late** – If you do, your adrenaline and cortisol levels will still be sky high at bedtime. If that evening turbo session is unavoidable, wait and go to bed an hour later, until you feel that 'sleep pressure' build (increasing feeling of drowsiness) as these hormones gradually fade in the bloodstream.
- **Eat dinner at least two hours before bedtime** – This will give your body time to digest. And resist that glass of wine. Even a glass or two can interfere with sleep, particularly the REM part.
- **We love our coffee but forgo the late-afternoon brew** – Caffeine makes us feel alert by blocking the receptors of adenosine. The effects of this build up during the day, creating a mounting feeling of sleepiness. You may be a fast caffeine metaboliser, meaning you can down an after-dinner espresso without consequence, but caffeine is still floating around in most people's bloodstreams for a good six hours.
- **Ensure your room is cool (18–20ºC/64–68ºF)** – Some pro teams have even experimented with supplying their riders with cooling mattress toppers containing a network of tubes in which cold water flows. Us mortals could just turn off the radiator in the bedroom and open a window.
- **Create a super dark bedroom and avoid bedtime screen time** – Photo receptors in the eyes detect light and this may reduce the signals to the brain to release the sleepy hormone melatonin.

To recap: no nice frothy afternoon cappuccino, cosy duvet film-watching, late-night partying, curry or cheeky glasses of red. You're welcome.

Napping: aka 'the siesta for speed'

Napping has an image problem – think 'Nana nap' – but put the word 'power' in front of it and own it because it is the secret training weapon of the pro cyclist. It will help you train harder and recover faster. We're not talking about the involuntary post-ride, mid-afternoon comatose state here, but a strategically planned 20-minute daytime sleep. The ideal length is 20–30 minutes, as this means you'll still be in the first two stages of sleep (see 'Deciphering sleep data' below) so you won't feel too groggy on waking. Or sleep for the full 90-minute sleep cycle. But even a 10-minute nap has been shown to immediately improve cognitive performance and energy. 'Siesta for speed' anyone?

The nappuccino

Cyclists love coffee and napping. Combine your beloved caffeine fix with a nap and you have a combination made in heaven: the nappuccino. Caffeine takes 30 minutes to peak in the bloodstream. Drink your coffee, set a timer for 20 or 25 minutes. Nap. Rise alert and raring to go. Afternoon training session anyone? Just remember the alarm, because if you nap longer than 25 minutes you risk feeling sluggish, offsetting the gains from the caffeine kick.

Deciphering sleep data

So, you woke up today and checked your sleep data via your smart watch or wearable. It says you got 2 hours 53 minutes of REM, 5 hours and 42 minutes of light sleep, were awake for three minutes and had barely any deep sleep. What does it all mean? The language of sleep can be baffling, but if you're keen to decipher your sleep data, here's the essential low-down.

Basically, we move through a series of 90-minute sleep cycles every night. Each cycle has four stages. The first two are light sleep, totalling about 30 minutes. Stage three is slow-wave, or deep, sleep. This is where blood pressure and heart rate drop, muscle damage is repaired, and human growth hormone (HGH) is released. The last stage is REM sleep, which plays a role in memory consolidation and emotional processing.

Then the cycle begins again. Most of us need to sleep through five 90-minute cycles, which would take seven and a half hours, or six cycles, which equates to nine hours. The more cycles you can tick off, the perkier you'll feel. However, sleep experts have questioned the accuracy of wearable sleep tracking devices in comparison with a gold-standard polysomnography test performed in a lab, so take the data with a pinch of salt. It has been suggested that the only numbers that standard sleep tracking devices are pretty good at recording is how many hours you've slept, which, to be fair, is very useful as we tend to think we've slept longer than we have. They are a lot less accurate when it comes to deciphering stages like REM or deep sleep. You can test this yourself by wearing two different trackers on the same night and comparing the data on these stages. Yes, I have done this. Sad but true. Or ignore your negative sleep data, get up, layer on the Lycra and crack on regardless. That's what double espressos were invented for, right? Jokes aside, it is important to ensure you get the best possible night's sleep, so pay attention and try to follow the sleep hacks on p. 140.

FULL GAS FOREVER

Slowing down the breathing fast-tracks the body into sleep mode.

Sleep-inducing exercises

Don't want to pop pills to up your sleep score? There are simple exercises that engage the body's parasympathetic, or rest-and-digest, nervous system. They were in use in yoga eons before the invention of CBD gummies and are now backed by numerous studies. Slowing down the breathing fast-tracks the body into sleep mode by dialling down the opposing fight-or-flight state. This wired state could be a hangover from a packed day at the office when the body is flooded by adrenaline or cortisol, but slow breathing can also reduce the feelings of wakefulness that stem from a hard evening interval session if you're still bouncing off the walls at bedtime. You can also use visualisations, such as imagining different parts of the body feeling heavy. Anyone who has attended a yoga class will be familiar with this as 'relaxation' or Savasana in Sanskrit.

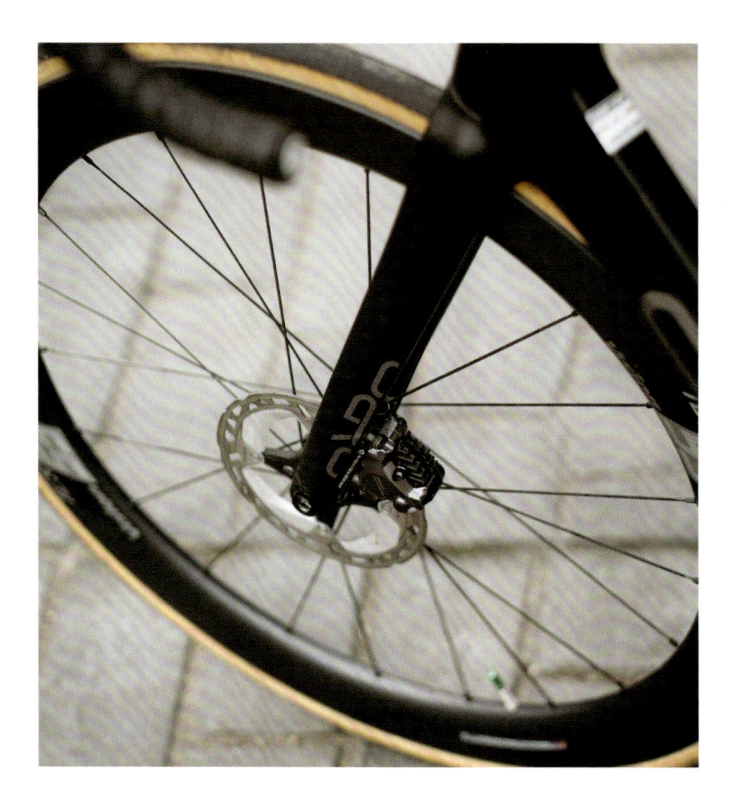

- **Circle breathing** – Visualise a circle. Start at the base of the circle and imagine breathing up one side to the top. As you exhale, visualise breathing down the other side until you get back to the base. Repeat 10 times.

Relaxation exercises

These relaxation exercises are based on visualising or systematically relaxing different parts of the body. Do them lying on a mat or in bed (as long as you are able to stay awake) with your legs bent or straight and your arms by your side, palms facing up.

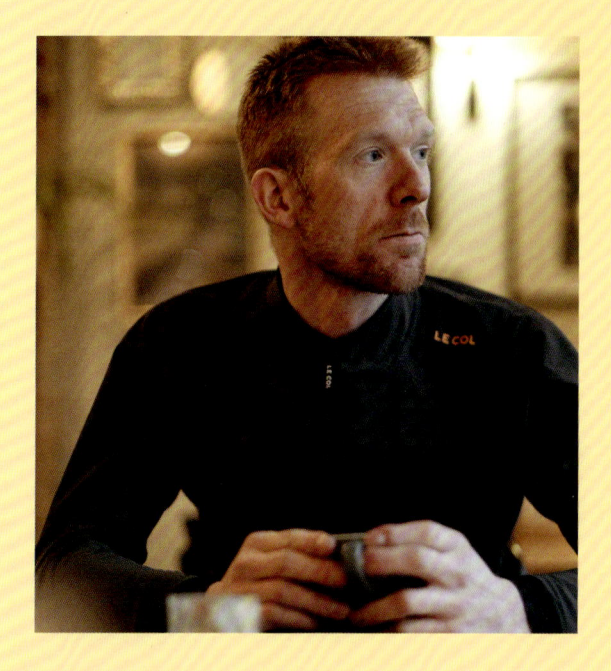

Breathing exercises

These techniques are best performed sitting up on a chair on in bed. They work well if done prior to a relaxation exercise (*see* right).

Chose one of these three breathing exercises to try:

- **Count the breath** – Inhale for one, two, three, four seconds, then exhale for one, two, three, four seconds. Repeat four times. Now increase the count by inhaling for five and exhaling for five. Repeat four times. Finally inhale for six and exhale for six. Repeat four times.
- **Hold the pause** – Take a slow, deep breath in and hold your breath at the top for a few seconds. Take a long slow breath out and hold again at the end of the exhalation. Repeat 10 times.

- **Heavy body** – Focus on your feet and imagine them becoming heavier. Now repeat the process as you move slowly up the body by focusing on the legs, hips, back, shoulders, arms and head.
- **Visualising a happy place** – Visualise a place where you felt most content or at ease – maybe somewhere you've been on holiday. Try to imagine the scene in as much detail as possible, including colours, smells and sounds.
- **Listening** – Try to listen to the sounds furthest away, such as the noise of a plane or distant traffic. Now listen to sounds a bit closer, immediately outside your house. Shift your focus to noises inside the house. Finish by cupping your hands over your ears and taking six slow, deep breaths, listening to your amplified breathing.

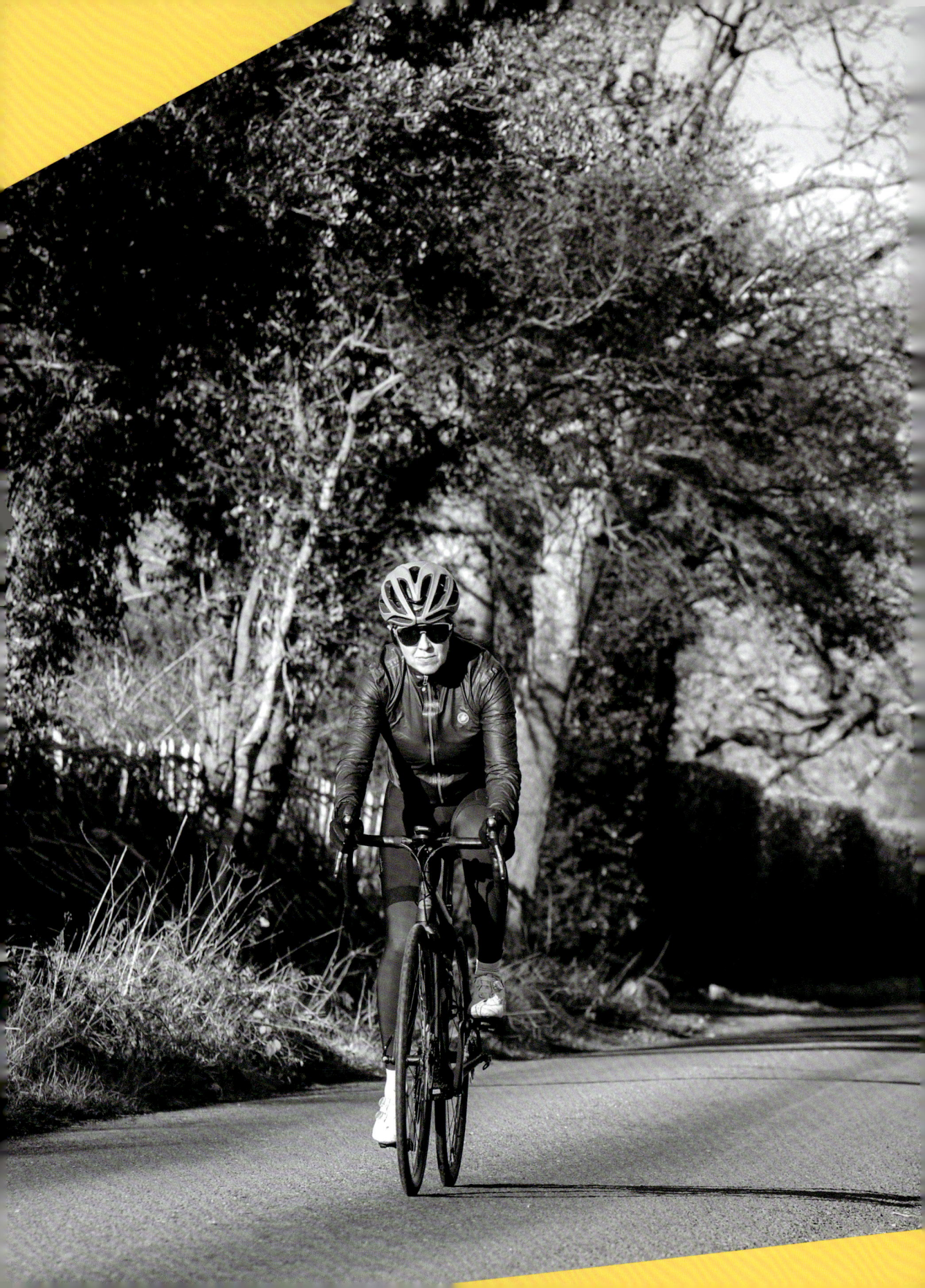

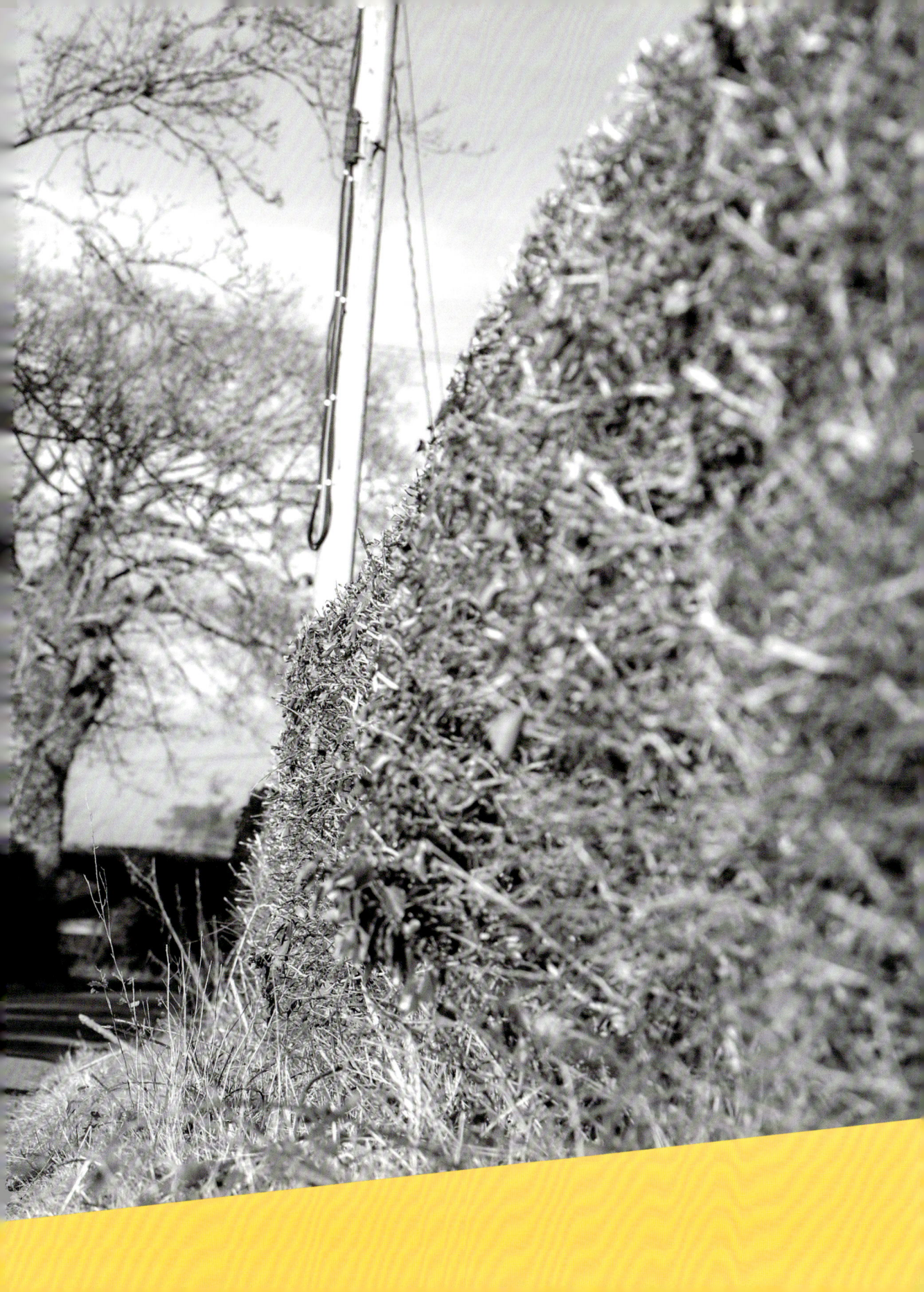

HORMONES

Lexie Williamson

Try not to get emotional, but we're going to talk about hormones: how they impact on your pedalling as you get older and what you can do about it. In particular, the big three that affect cycling performance – testosterone, human growth hormone and oestrogen, which female midlife riders may be all too painfully familiar with. It's going to be fine – I promise. Deep breath…

The midlife cyclist's guide to hormones

There are many hormones that affect performance, including melatonin, which plays a big role in sleep and, therefore, recovery. But first let's get the lowdown on the three biggies:

1) Testosterone

Testosterone does a number of things that are conducive to strong riding, including stimulating the production of red blood cells, increasing lean muscle mass, improving your ability to recover and increasing bone density. A blood test can reveal testosterone levels but after 30, levels decline at 1 per cent each year, meaning men have roughly half the testosterone in their 70s and 80s than they had in their 20s. In women, levels of testosterone decline between the ages of 20 and 40 but have plateaued out and are stable by menopause.

Testosterone supplementation also has its risks, including cardiovascular disease and prostate cancer for men.

Aside from taking supplementation, there are easy, less risky ways to boost your levels (*see* p.150). Ensure that you recover properly, as this spell off the bike will give your testosterone levels a boost and build your training slowly over time. For example, if you are currently training five hours a week but want to increase this to 15 hours, just add an hour of training a week at a time, being sure to add a recovery week in every three to four weeks, until you reach the desired volume.

Something else that should be done gradually, so as not to mess with normal hormonal function, is weight loss. Shed the pounds gradually over time and continue to consume sufficient calories to fuel your rides and other exercise. It is possible to negatively affect testosterone levels by being too lean. Think what weight you performed your best at rather than falling into the trap of always believing that lighter is faster. Finally, testosterone levels are highest in the morning for both men and women – a good argument for pulling on the Lycra and getting out there early.

Long rides can deplete testosterone

While we may feel pumped up after a ride, studies have actually shown that 90 minutes of submaximal exercise results in a slight decrease in testosterone, while exercise of moderate to hard intensity for over two hours results in a significant decrease. Over the course of a three-week grand tour the testosterone of pro cyclists will drop each week. This drop is linked not just to the physical muscular activity, but also to metabolic stress, which induces fatigue in many of the systems that control hormone levels. This could be down to a few factors: elevated cortisol levels, consuming too few calories for the energy required for the workout and changes in luteinising hormone, which helps to create testosterone. This actually may not affect performance – after all, the pros seem to do OK – but it's something to keep an eye on. If you are experiencing symptoms like persistent fatigue or loss of libido then you've definitely gone out too long, too hard and too often, and it is probably affecting your testosterone levels, so ease off a little.

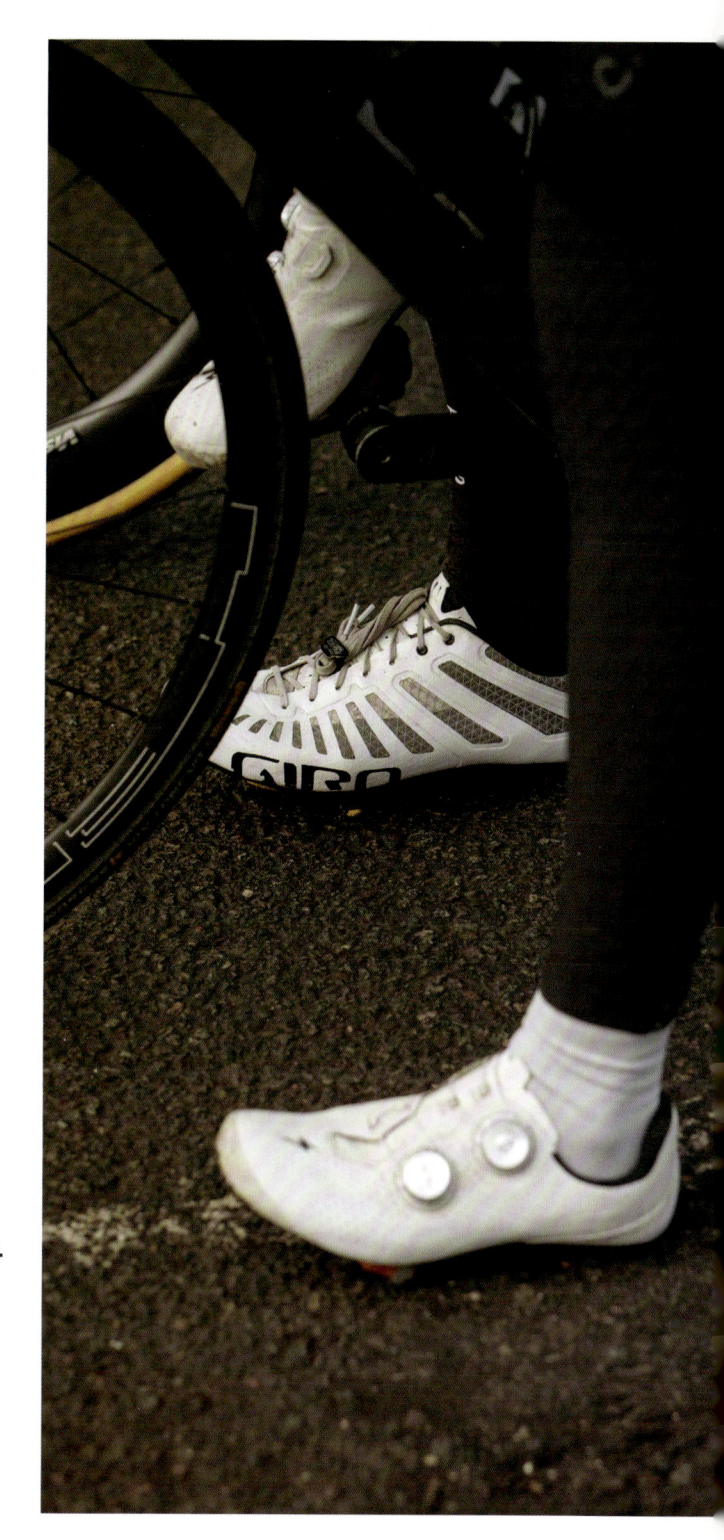

Another way to counter the long rides is to boost testosterone levels with weight training. Some coaches even recommend Masters cyclists split the week between 80 per cent riding and 20 per cent strength work. Technically, it doesn't actually have to involve lifting weights; bodyweight or plyometric (quick jumping-type exercises) will also increase levels. Try squats to recruit the major muscle groups like the glutes and quads or other resistance training classics such as hand release press-ups (*see* p.31) and Planks, *see* Forearm Plank, p.44.

2) Oestrogen

Important for bone health for both sexes, oestrogen levels have a huge impact on female cyclists by influencing power output, increasing feel-good chemicals like dopamine and serotonin, and improving reaction times. As any female midlife cyclist knows, you hit the perimenopause and things can change, dramatically. Around the age of 40 your ovaries produce less oestrogen and progesterone. In fact, it is common to experience a 10-fold decrease in oestrogen compared to levels experienced during certain phases of the menstrual cycle. As hormone levels drop you may see an accumulation in belly fat and experience the loss of lean muscle mass – not ideal for a lean, mean cyclist! But here's the good news: a study of 48 women aged 55 to 72 found that the group of women who exercised for three hours a week showed a significant drop in menopausal symptoms like fatigue and insomnia compared to the group that were largely sedentary. The active group also reported better mood and mental well-being.

The message is loud and clear: get out there and ride even if it seems like a struggle to drag that Lycra on. Strength training is also essential, partly because your risk of osteoporosis rises sharply in this stage of life and cycling doesn't build bone density. Strength training also boosts the muscle power that you are in danger of losing in perimenopause. Don't skimp on ride nutrition and end up under-fuelling, and hydrate well, especially if you are riding

> **A study of 48 women aged 55 to 72 found that the group of women who exercised for three hours a week showed a significant drop in menopausal symptoms like fatigue and insomnia compared to the group that were largely sedentary.**

in hot weather and suffer with hot flushes so are already struggling with your body temperature. You could try pre-hydrating with a sodium-rich drink before you ride, then ensure you consume one bottle per hour on the bike and drink a protein-rich recovery drink when you're done.

Are you getting enough protein?
Perimenopausal and menopausal cyclists (and all cyclists from midlife and older) should ensure they get sufficient protein in their diet. This is around 90g (3oz) per day. Unsure what the recommended amount looks like? It's more than you think and reading this list you may realise that you've been under-consuming protein for years. Go for whole-food sources such as eggs, lean meat, dairy or poultry if you are not vegan or vegetarian. Here are some examples of the protein content of everyday foods:

- Greek yogurt – 15g (½oz) protein
- Two eggs – 12g (⅖oz) protein
- Half a cup of oats – 5g (⅙oz) protein
- 30g nuts – 5g (⅙oz) protein
- A standard can of tuna – 27g (1oz) protein

Vegan? Try peanut butter (two tablespoons = 7g/¼oz protein), a scoop of protein powder (20g/⅔oz protein) or 30g/1oz nuts (5g/⅙oz protein) as well as tofu, lentils or black beans. For more advice on protein (and all things cycling and diet), turn to chapter 13.

3) Human growth hormone (HGH)
HGH, or simply 'growth hormone', decreases from its peak levels in puberty by 1–2 per cent every year from the age of 30, and for the rest of our lives, according to Phil Cavell, author of *The Midlife Cyclist*. The hormone, which is secreted in the pituitary gland, essentially makes us bigger and stronger, and the natural decline of it with age can lead to a reduction in aerobic capacity, a decrease in lean muscle bulk and an increase in body fat, especially around the middle. Unfortunately, there are side effects to taking synthetic HGH or we'd all be wolfing it down. It's definitely not a route to your former, stronger cycling self that is worth pursuing.

It is thought, though, that there are more natural ways to slow the inevitable decline of HGH. These include getting plenty of sleep in the first half of the night when your HGH production is highest, replacing refined carbs with healthy fats like nuts, olive oil and avocado and, yes – the two solid training foundations we keep returning to: high-intensity training sessions, which ramp up the heart rate, and lifting weights.

FULL GAS FOREVER

We need to modify our training regime as we age to maximise hormone balance by incorporating adequate rest time between sessions.

Simple ways to fight age-related hormone decline

So why are we not just popping testosterone, oestrogen and HGH pills like there's no tomorrow? Unfortunately, as already mentioned, there can be serious side effects to taking supplements. Luckily, there are a few more natural, common-sense and very achievable ways to boost the level of some of these hormones that affect riding performance but decline with age. Phil Cavell has written a list of behavioural changes that are all easily adopted to boost levels of some of these hormones.

- **Start resistance training** – This boosts production of both HGH and testosterone, and offsets weight gain and muscle loss. Cavell recommends dropping one or two bike sessions a week in favour of structured resistance training.
- **Get better sleep** – This is easier said than done as our levels of melatonin drop as we age, but managing a good sleep balance increases the production of HGH and testosterone. Try avoiding alcohol (known to disrupt REM) and sugar (especially at the end of the day).
- **Reduce sugar intake** – Cavell states that HGH levels are glucose sensitive. Reducing sugar will offset insulin sensitivity changes and help HGH production levels.
- **Monitor vitamin D levels** – Low levels of the vitamin are thought to be associated with inhibited testosterone production. The 'sunshine vitamin' also helps the body absorb calcium, is thought to be important for boosting the immune system and could possibly have a role in muscle contractions.
- **Reduce stress** – Stress releases the hormone cortisol, which inhibits the production of testosterone, oestrogen and progesterone. This stress can be related to everyday work pressures or other life stresses off the bike, but also overtraining with a lack of adequate recovery. To the body, they are both perceived as stress; it can't decipher the difference.
- **Don't skimp on recovery** – We need to modify our training regime as we age to maximise hormone balance by incorporating adequate rest time between sessions. 'Doing the same as we always have will embed fatigue, and negative metabolic and hormonal dynamics,' says Cavell. For more advice on recovery turn to chapter 14.

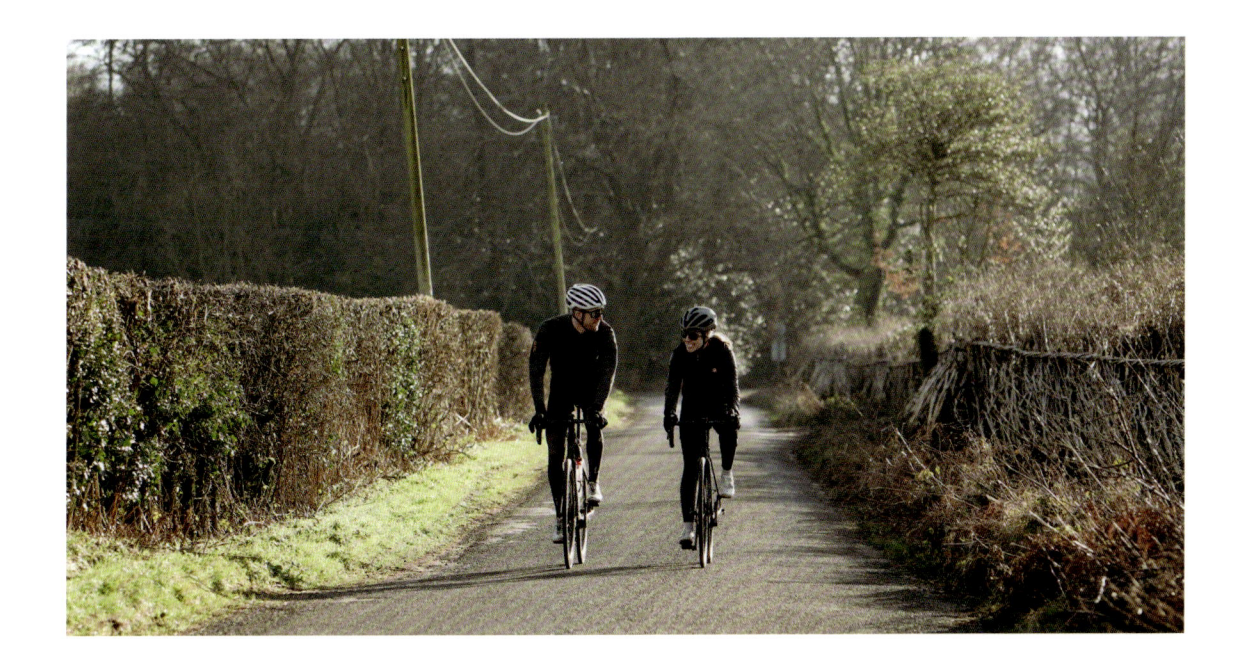

Interval, intervals, intervals

It's fine to enjoy long, steady rides as a Masters cyclist, but a 30–60-minute hard interval session will do wonders to increase levels of hormones like testosterone and HGH, and counter the decline in muscle mass experienced by both men and women. This makes it a good alternative to strength training for those allergic to the gym, although doing both is the gold standard. Think power and speed, power and speed. Workouts should be performed at over 80 per cent of your max heart rate in order to maintain a solid aerobic capacity. However, let's insert a common-sense caveat here: if you are overtraining and suffering with symptoms such as fatigue, don't try to squeeze in a hard interval session as it's highly unlikely to increase your testosterone levels and will just make you more tired.

Are you in love with cycling?

Ever reached the end of ride, turned to your cycling group and said: 'I loved that ride.' Well, it turns out that might be a more accurate statement than you realise. Scientists have found that alongside dopamine and other feel-good chemicals, the body releases the love hormone oxytocin, otherwise known as the 'cuddle chemical', when we exercise. Researchers found that levels of oxytocin, which is released when we fall in love or bond with our newborn baby, rose after subjects completed a 4 x 4 high-intensity interval workout on exercise bikes. Oxytocin promotes feelings of trust, relaxation and psychological stability. So, it's not your imagination: you really are obsessed with cycling.

GOING OFF-ROAD

Ed Clancy

Go on, get muddy and explore the great outdoors! Mountain biking, gravel riding and cyclo-cross are great training variations, ideal for mastering bike handling and a fun alternative to the road.

It's a common sight to see top road riders venturing off-road, especially in the winter months. Many of them, like Marianne Vos and Mathieu van der Poel, grew up riding mountain bikes or racing cyclo-cross. Other road riders adapt easily to the blossoming gravel racing scene, where roadies Matej Mohorič and Kasia Niewiadoma were both recent world champions.

So often our roads are busy and it's difficult to find your own space among a constant flow of cars, traffic lights and junctions. Paths, bridleways and tracks can provide a place of sanctuary, where many of the stresses of road riding disappear. Off-road riding, whether it is on muddy tracks, gravel roads or over wild terrain, is a totally different experience to road cycling. And yet, they share enough characteristics (yes, essentially two wheels and a chainset) to provide valuable training opportunities for road riders.

Off-road disciplines offer variety, especially for those zone 1 or 2 training rides, which can get pretty boring. They provide a chance to leave your comfort zone and enjoy a new stimulation to freshen up your training programme. You get to enjoy the feeling of escape, go deep into natural environments, learn new skills and, most of all, have some fun.

Mountain biking

Mountain biking is the most popular of the off-road disciplines. It has a totally different vibe to road riding. On the forest tracks, fun and adrenaline highs provide the buzz more than the serious competitive nature of the road. It's not about data – power, heart rates or speed – but the challenges and thrills or the terrain. And it is not so much about marginal gains as technical ability: you are too busy studying the path ahead to check your power output.

There are different race disciplines within mountain biking: the most dangerous is downhill, which is pure descent (usually from a high point accessed by ski lift or vehicle), while the energy-sapping enduro includes (usually

GOING OFF-ROAD

Bike handling skills are one of the biggest bonuses you will take back to the road from mountain biking.

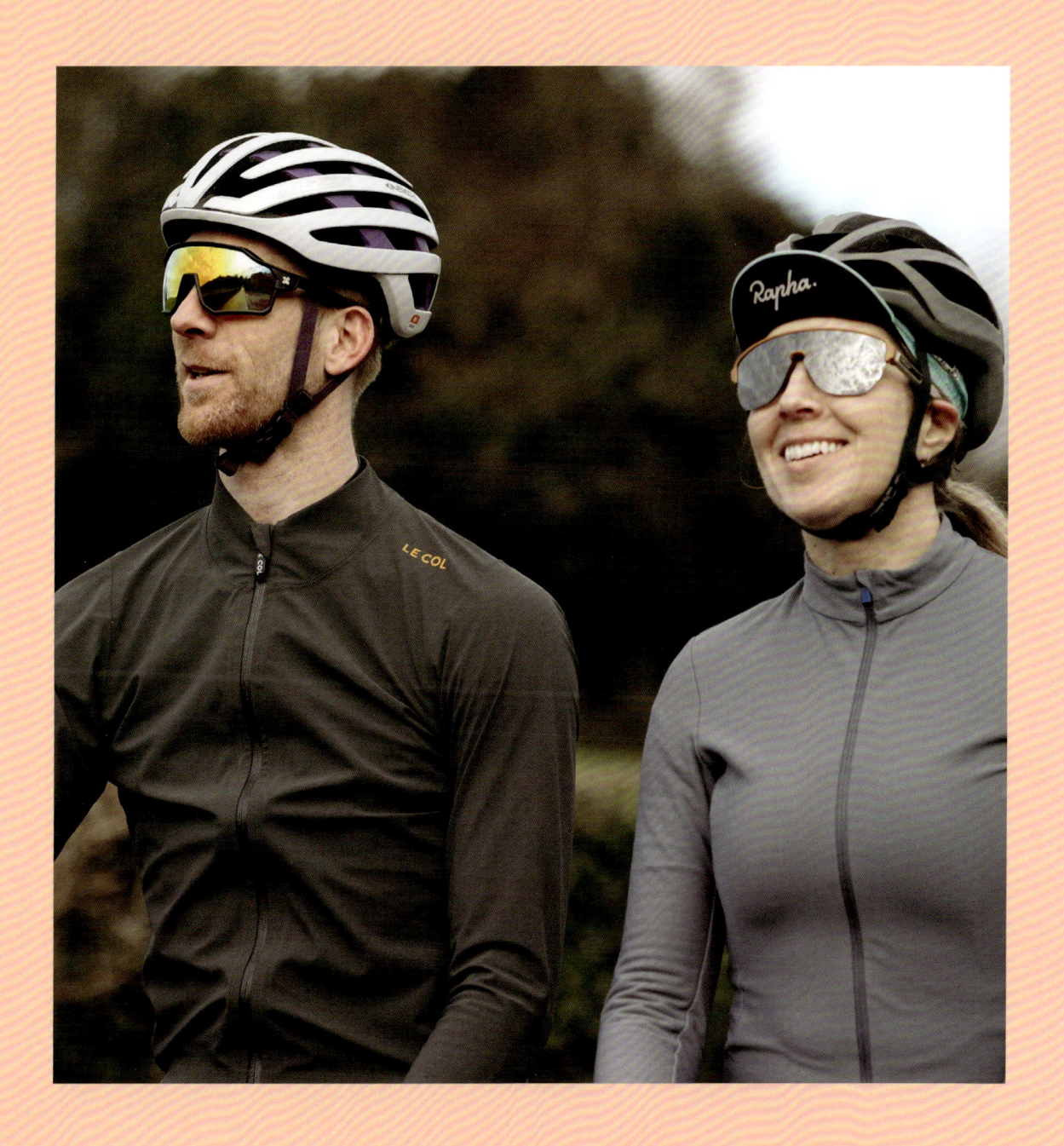

FULL GAS FOREVER

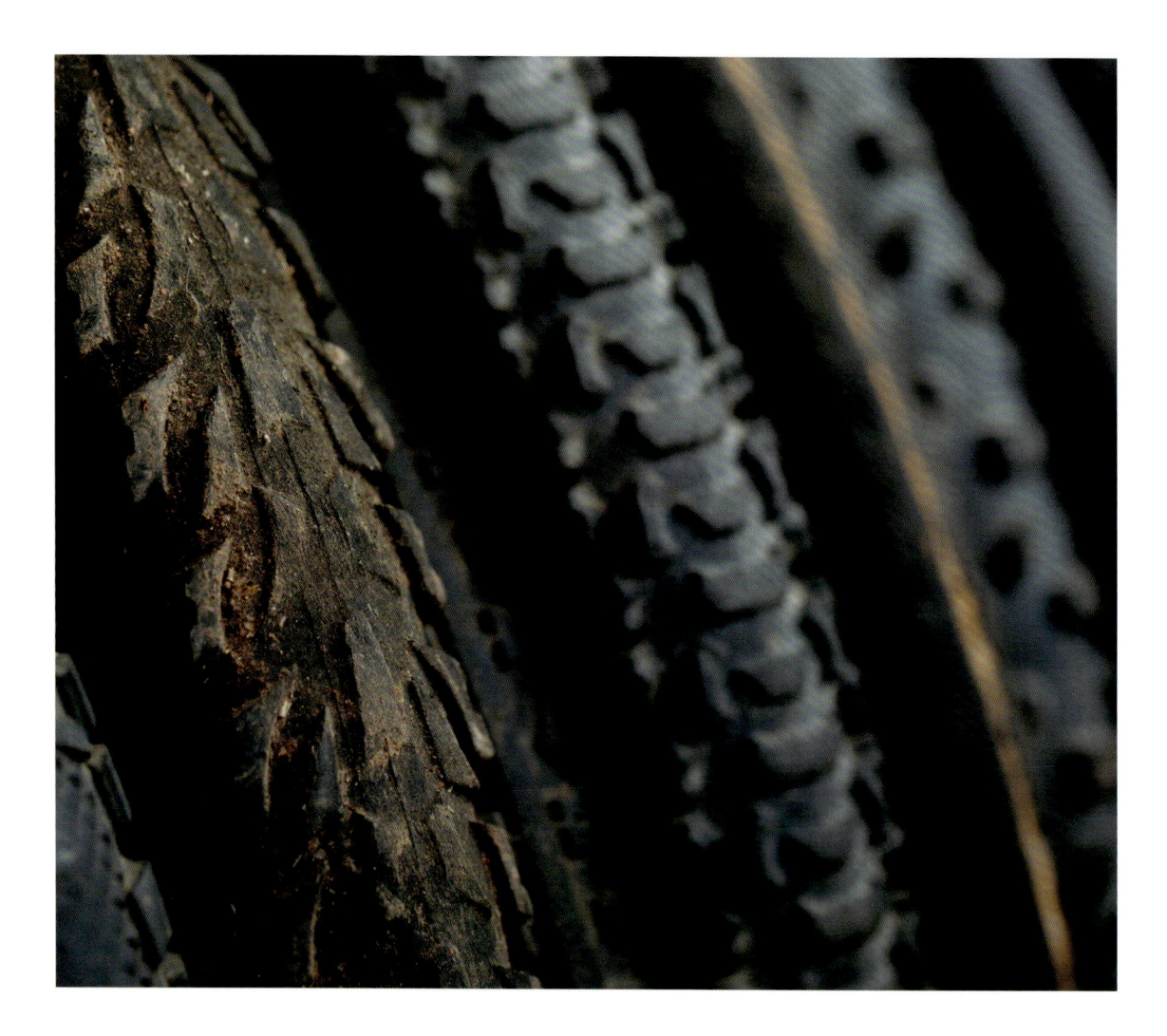

untimed) uphill rides between descents. Most people will ride cross-country through forest paths, single tracks and trails. They usually have some short, brutal climbs, tricky descents and a host of natural obstacles.

Even a fairly experienced road rider will find the bikes need a little getting used to. Mountain bikes will generally have an upright geometry front and rear suspension, wide handlebars and, although the wheels might have a similar width, the tyres will be fat with thick treads and tubes inflated to only 22–24psi. Riding style is necessarily different. A road cyclist can spend hours in the same position, but the MTB rider is constantly adjusting the bike and body for balance and navigating the terrain.

The ground can slip and slide beneath you or you find yourself on undulating ground with constant bumps and drops. You soon learn to be looser and become flexible on the bike. Mountain biking is a proper physical sport, an all-body workout using your upper body and arms so much more than on a road bike. It will do wonders for your core stability, strengthening the muscles that hold your spine and pelvis in place – something that will result in more stable and balanced positioning when you are back on your road bike.

Bike handling skills are one of the biggest bonuses you will take back to the road from mountain biking. The tracks are full of roots and ruts, rocks and trees, as well as sharp corners and sudden short climbs. Tackling these at pace might seem like something you are unlikely to need on a B-road in Lincolnshire, but they are skills that are just as handy for evading potholes or fallen bidons, keeping your balance on slippery surfaces or finding a gap in a bunch sprint.

Cornering on descents is a critical part of mountain biking, with uneven switchbacks and tight corners a regular occurrence on many trails. The skills you gain from picking a line, judging when to brake going into the bend, how far to lean into the bend and when to accelerate out will enhance your ability and your confidence when negotiating tougher corners at greater speed on the road. Going up has benefits as well. Those high-intensity sessions on a trainer are often difficult to replicate on the road, but they have a natural equivalent on the trails. Most courses are full of short, steep hills that require brief but explosive bursts of power, especially if it's a heavy slog up a muddy hill.

You learn to use your gears effectively on these courses. Because the terrain quickly changes – and so does your speed – it's imperative that you're looking ahead and anticipating the correct gear to be in to maintain a steady cadence. Generally you will get by riding in the wrong gear on the road, but the terrain here is unforgiving. Fortunately, mountain bikes have pretty low gears and can help you get up virtually anything. Get it wrong, though, and you can be left pushing a heavy bike up the hill.

Your focus changes too on a mountain bike. One of the fundamental skills of mountain biking is keeping your eyes up and scanning the trail ahead. If you are looking down at your front wheel, that gnarly root will appear out of nowhere. If you've clocked it from a distance, you will have time to calculate the best way to approach it and negotiate it. This is another habit that will be useful when you are back on the road.

There is one downside: there's a pretty good chance you will fairly regularly fall off the bike one way or another when mountain biking. I reckon I crash, fall or have a close escape once every 10 rides or so. But there is a difference between falling in a muddy ditch at 16km/h (10mph) and losing your front wheel on a road at 55km/h (35mph). You invariably get up and get back on. Coming off is part of the sport and usually it's really not that bad. So, on the plus side, you are getting used to falling, maybe learning something about landing well, and won't be so fearful next time.

All these skills are transferable to road cycling and although they may be needed in less extreme situations or in a different context, they will give you the confidence to ride braver and better. You can't buy that kind of boost. Knowing you have the technique to deal with situations –

cornering on descents, dealing with unexpected terrain or weather or negotiating obstacles – allows you to ride faster and stronger. Any time spent out in the forests and hills definitely won't be wasted and I can almost guarantee it'll be a lot more fun than an 80km (50-mile) zone 2 ride on unchallenging roads.

Electric mountain bikes

Electric bikes can be a real boon to the recreational cyclist, but are of little help to the keen road cyclist. The 25km/h (15.5mph) limiter means any assistance gained isn't worth the extra weight. However, off-road is a different story. When you are out in the woods and trails, you rarely hit 25km/h (15.5mph). The development of electric mountain bikes (e-MTBs) has been a game-changer here. If you think it's cheating, ask yourself what mountain biking is all about. For a start, you can pedal an e-MTB just as hard as an analogue bike – you just go further and faster – so the effort you exert is a choice. The fun is in negotiating gnarly paths, tricky descents and high banks, not cycling for 15 minutes along a track to get there or the energy-sapping muddy climb to the top of the hill. With electric assistance, you even get to try the steep, tricky climbs that you would otherwise be wheeling the bike up. The downsides? They are slightly heavier and they are not cheap, but if you get a chance, I'd really recommend giving electric a go.

Cyclo-cross

Cyclo-cross began as a way for road racers to add some variety to their off-season training, but is now a year-round sport in its own right. For those roadies missing the element of competition and speed in their winter training, cyclo-cross might be the answer. Just like mountain biking, cyclo-cross relies on technical skills, but it is also super-frantic, fast and punchy, requiring explosive short, sharp efforts and a whole lot of stamina.

> **For those roadies missing the element of competition and speed in their winter training, cyclo-cross might be the answer.**

GOING OFF-ROAD

The gravel scene has been built on inclusivity. It has a reputation for being welcoming and non-judgemental about bikes or ability, with elite riders and novices starting together.

Cyclo-cross races are usually short – lasting 40–60 minutes – and are ridden over around 10 laps of mixed terrain (so you never get obviously left behind as you would on the road) with various obstacles placed en route. Cyclo-cross bikes resemble road bikes, but with forks and stays providing more clearance for wider tyres and mud. If you are racing for fun you can use a mountain bike, but don't expect to win. In good weather or in summer you can get away with using an old road bike with wider tyres.

All those bike handling skills that featured in mountain biking come into play here with the added stress of racing. It can be a steep learning curve – including perfecting your bunny hops over hurdles, running with your bike on your shoulder or slogging through a sand pit – but it's all fantastic fun.

Significantly, cyclo-cross differs from the road in that it is an individual sport. Closer to time trialling than road racing, it is what they call 'character building'. There's very little opportunity to draft (or for someone else to suck your wheel), but that means assessing your own capabilities, practising self-control and sticking to your own pace. If you ride cyclo-cross in the winter, you'll face hail, snow, mud, wind and cold, and come summer you'll be so used to it that you can leave the rainy day whining to those who spent chunks of the off-season in Majorca.

Gravel racing

If all this seems a bit too close to nature, but you still want to escape the traffic and tarmac, then gravel might be the answer. Gravel racing is basically – and sometimes literally – going off-road on a road bike. It shares the transferable skills of mountain biking and cyclo-cross, including bike handing, resilience, flexibility and whole-body strength, but with less of the extreme terrain and challenging obstacles.

Gravel bikes have a longer wheelbase and a taller headtube that lets the rider sit more upright, and low gearing options, but for someone riding infrequently it is possible to change to wider wheels on your road bike (preferably not your best one) and use that. Alternatively, some buy a gravel bike and swap to narrower tyres for training on the road, taking advantage of the extra road work on a heavier, slower bike.

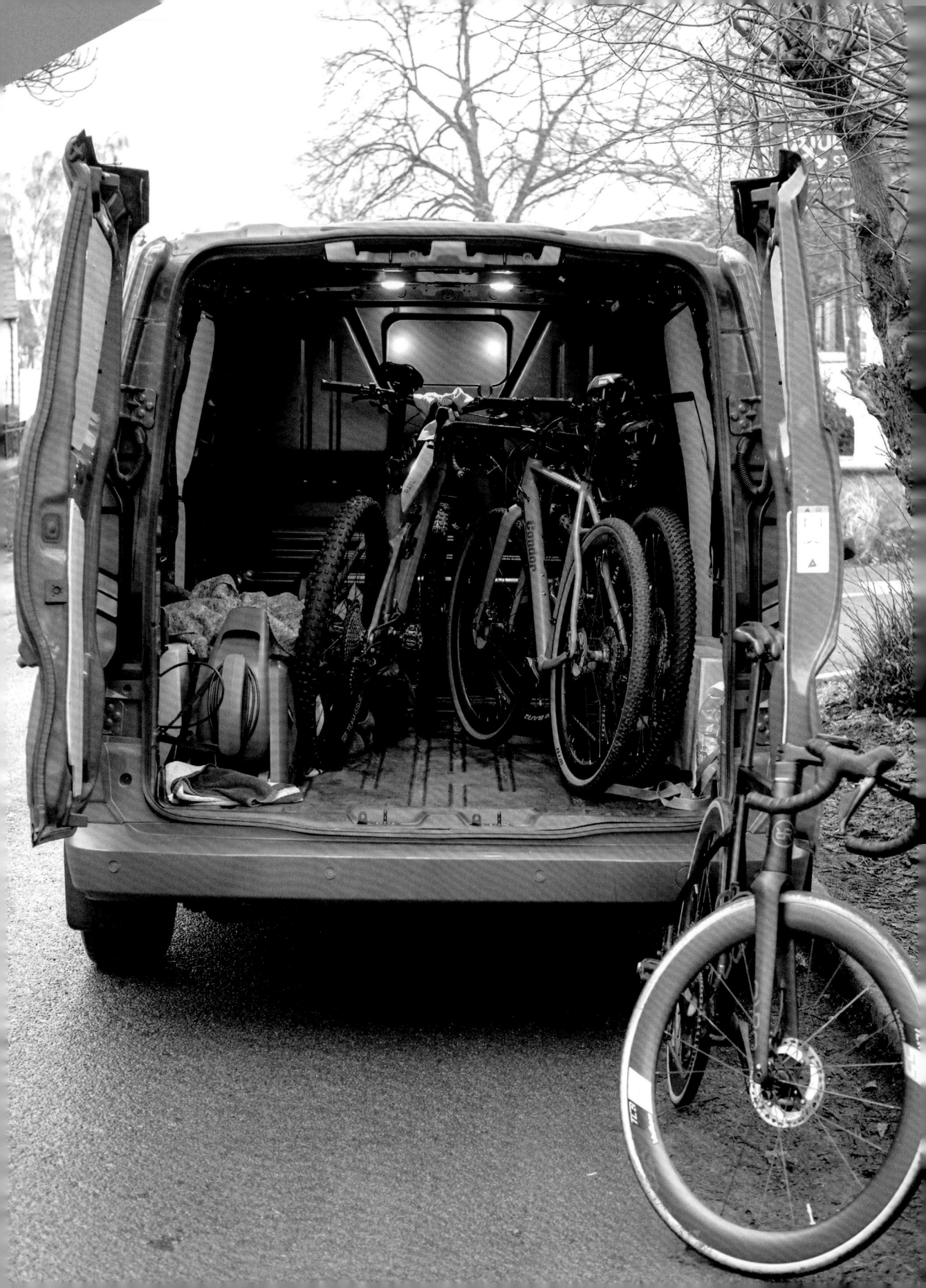

You are not just riding on gravel paths; the name 'adventure cycling' is more apt as routes also take you on single tracks, canal towpaths, bridleways and other terrains. Races and rides are often endurance-based distances familiar to road riders with distances ranging from 40 to 320km (25 to 200 miles) – and are obviously slower-paced.

Gravel riding has taken off over the last decade or so, not least because of cyclists turning from the road for training or because they prefer the car- and regulation-free environment. The gravel scene has been built on inclusivity. It has a reputation for being welcoming and non-judgemental about bikes or ability, with elite riders and novices starting together. And despite it having the solo characteristics of cyclo-cross, there is usually an 'in-it-together' attitude along the route.

Gravel riding has taken off over the last decade or so, not least because of cyclists turning from the road for training or because they prefer the car- and regulation-free environment.

I grew up riding mountain bikes off-road as a child and that feeling of freedom, exploration and escape has never left me. Everything about the road (or even more so, track) bike is built for competition. The geometry, lightness and precision of the bike is all directed to speed. Off the road, the bike is a different beast. It is resilient, upright, practical; it is built for survival. Does it help your road riding? You bet.

I was a pretty terrible road rider, but I won criterium races against riders who aerobically were stronger than me. Because I was comfortable on my bike, I could hang with them and had the advantage when it came to taking corners at speed. It was a comfort born of riding through forests on paths of mud, dodging tree stumps and going round bends without losing my back wheel.

Years later, I find myself riding sportives where hundreds of the riders really struggle. They are fit enough, have trained well, but they either lack the confidence in their riding or the skills to deal with anything technically challenging, such as a pothole or a moving bollard. These are the kind of things that come naturally when you are used to riding off-road. So, what's to lose? You won't become a worse rider and there's much to be gained. And, you never know, you might even discover you prefer it!

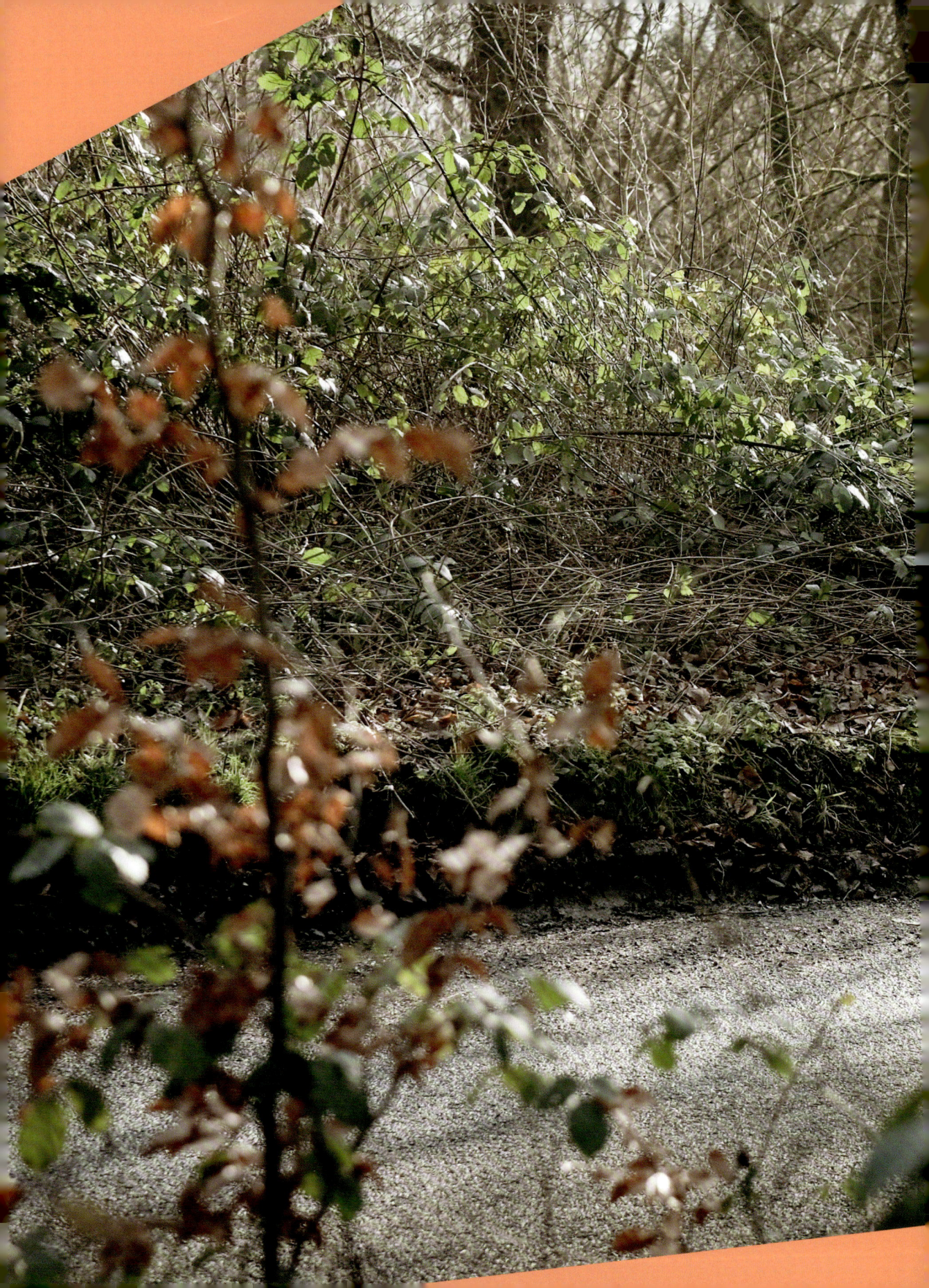

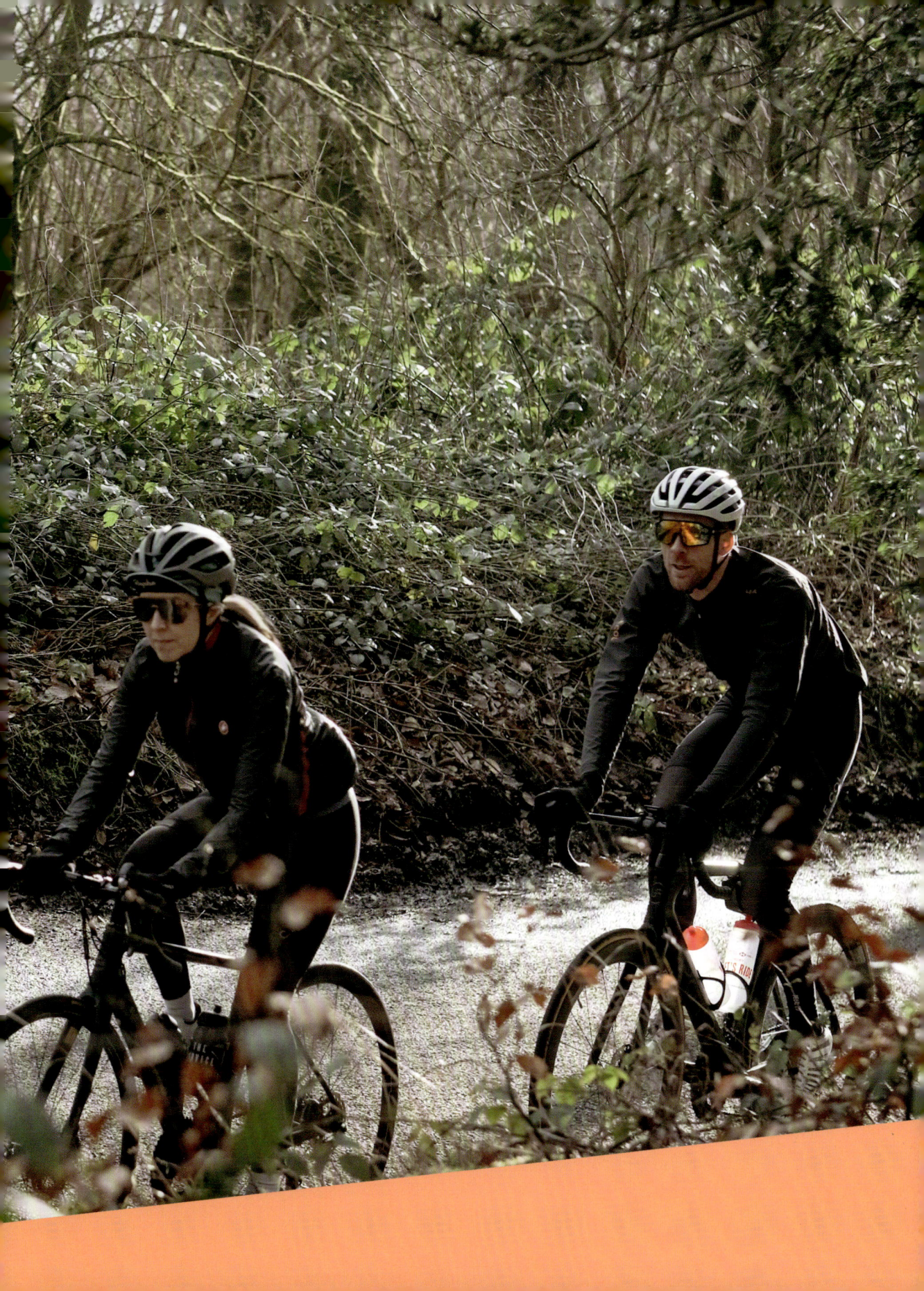

INDOOR TRAINING

Ed Clancy

Turbos, rollers and other indoor trainers are a perfect solution for fair-weather or time-pressed cyclists, but increasingly make for an effective element of training, too. Here's the lowdown on what they are and how to use them.

I don't believe there is anything better than being out on the open road, but indoor cycling has its own distinct advantages in that it is convenient, great for getting maximum training value from limited time, and, it has to be said, can often be great fun and even sociable. An indoor option is always worth having, not just for when there is ice on the roads or if your time is squeezed, but also when you are ready for focused training. It is much easier to monitor your output and cadence without having to deal with traffic lights, cars and external influences.

The sweat room

Where to put the thing. Many trainers are foldable and portable (*see* below), but who really wants to have to get them out and set them up every time they need a quick session of intervals – especially if you are using your bike, too? The ideal is for the trainer to have a dedicated space in the garage, shed or basement away from distractions and people to irritate. I leave mine set up through most of the winter. If that isn't always possible, then being able to move it a short distance to the corner of the room is the next best thing. The more difficult it is to jump on and start pedalling, the less incentive there is to use it.

The first thing you notice when you start indoor training is the sweat. The amount of heat you generate without being outdoors in the fresh air is incredible. No matter if you are the most naturally fragrant person, after a few minutes of hard work the drops will appear and they won't stop. If you are not careful, you will stink the house out. Even in winter. So the number one requirement is a fan – not some flimsy office one but a big industrial machine. It pays to have a towel handily placed too – you can usually drape it over the handlebars – so you can grab it easily to wipe yourself down. And think of the carpet. That sweat will rain down so get a washable mat to put the trainer on.

That amount of sweat means you will need water, too. Unlike being on the road, it can be unlimited, so have as many bottles to hand as you need. You want to avoid getting up and going to fill up after every set. It's pretty likely that you will be using your phone or a laptop to monitor your effort, so they need to be visible, too. A phone can be attached to the bars easily enough, but a laptop will need a stand or a table.

Types of trainer

There are various options open to those looking to train indoors. Which one you plump for is largely down to your budget, the amount of space you have available, and your personal comfort and convenience.

The traditional option of rollers is the cheapest and easiest of them, with the advantage of often being foldable and transportable, which helps with storage. You ride your own bike on rotating drums and once you have got used to them they offer a good imitation of road riding, so help with balance and bike handling skills, although the only way you can modify your power is by changing gear.

A static bike – a version of the gym fitness bikes – is a bulky and permanently set-up option. The cheaper end of the market allows for little more than general fitness, but high-end stationary bikes have taken them to another level. They are quieter, have sophisticated resistance mechanisms and provide more than enough data. The best ones go some way to replicating the experience of a road bike. It isn't your bike so you don't wear it out, which is an advantage, but it will never feel quite like the one you are used to riding outdoors.

A mid-priced turbo (budget versions are seriously noisy) can provide the best of both these worlds. They are designed to take any road bikes (and many hybrid or mountain bikes) and can be 'wheel-on', where the rear wheel of your bike is mounted on a roller that uses fluid or magnets to generate resistance, or 'direct-drive', where the wheel is removed and replaced by a cassette that is driven by your drivetrain. Both of them use your own bike (although special rear tyres are recommended for the hard-wearing wheel-on turbos), and are usually foldable and easily stored.

Indoor cycling has its own distinct advantages in that it is convenient, great for getting maximum training value from limited time, and, it has to be said, can often be great fun and even sociable.

Set-up and posture

If you are fitting your outdoor bike on to your trainer you should not need to adjust the set-up. It is worth checking the bike is level or a centimetre higher, as sometimes the front wheel is lower when positioned in a trainer. You can put the wheel in a riser or even use a book to raise it if necessary. The turbo will highlight any problems with your set-up as you tend to remain static on it, whereas when riding outdoors you are constantly adjusting position, which can hide some issues.

The main difference in posture is that your grip on the handlebars is less important. When you feel like it, you can sit bolt upright and take your hands off the bars, riding with your chest back, stretching the spine, and relaxing your shoulders and elbows. However, bear in mind that your static position and the fact that the resistance will prevent you from freewheeling will mean you become fatigued sooner. Don't be shy of taking a rest and starting afresh.

Trainer tips

- Take your time to build up fitness. There's no need to go all-out on every session.
- Limit yourself to two short and sweet sessions a week – 30–60 minutes will be enough.
- Warming up properly will enable you to get the best out of each session.
- Change the gears and the turbo's resistance level to vary your cadence and effort.
- Don't forget to eat and drink.

Trainer workouts

There are plenty of different workouts available with many of the apps providing drills for cadence, sprints and other skills, as well as programmes focusing on different goals and disciplines. Here are a few examples to use in sessions. The number of reps stated are just guidance, so work up to them if necessary: intensity is more important than quantity.

30–30s

Sometimes called Billats (designed by French exercise physiologist Veronique Billat), these call for 30 seconds at 100 per cent of your FTP followed by 30 seconds at an easy recovery rate (of course, for much of your rest time your metabolism is still operating at near 100 per cent). Begin with 5–10 minutes and work up to three sets of 10 bursts with a full recovery between each set. These aren't difficult if you stick to FTP and you might be amazed how quickly your fitness improves after just a short amount of time.

Tabata

Doctor Izumi Tabata's intervals are great for the time-challenged rider or to finish off a session, as they are short and even more intense than 30–30s. They comprise intervals of 20 seconds at full gas followed by just 10 seconds of rest and can be your whole workout. They can be extremely difficult, so begin the intervals at 100 watts or so above FTP and take it from there. The sets can also be repeated up to four times with a two- or three-minute rest between each.

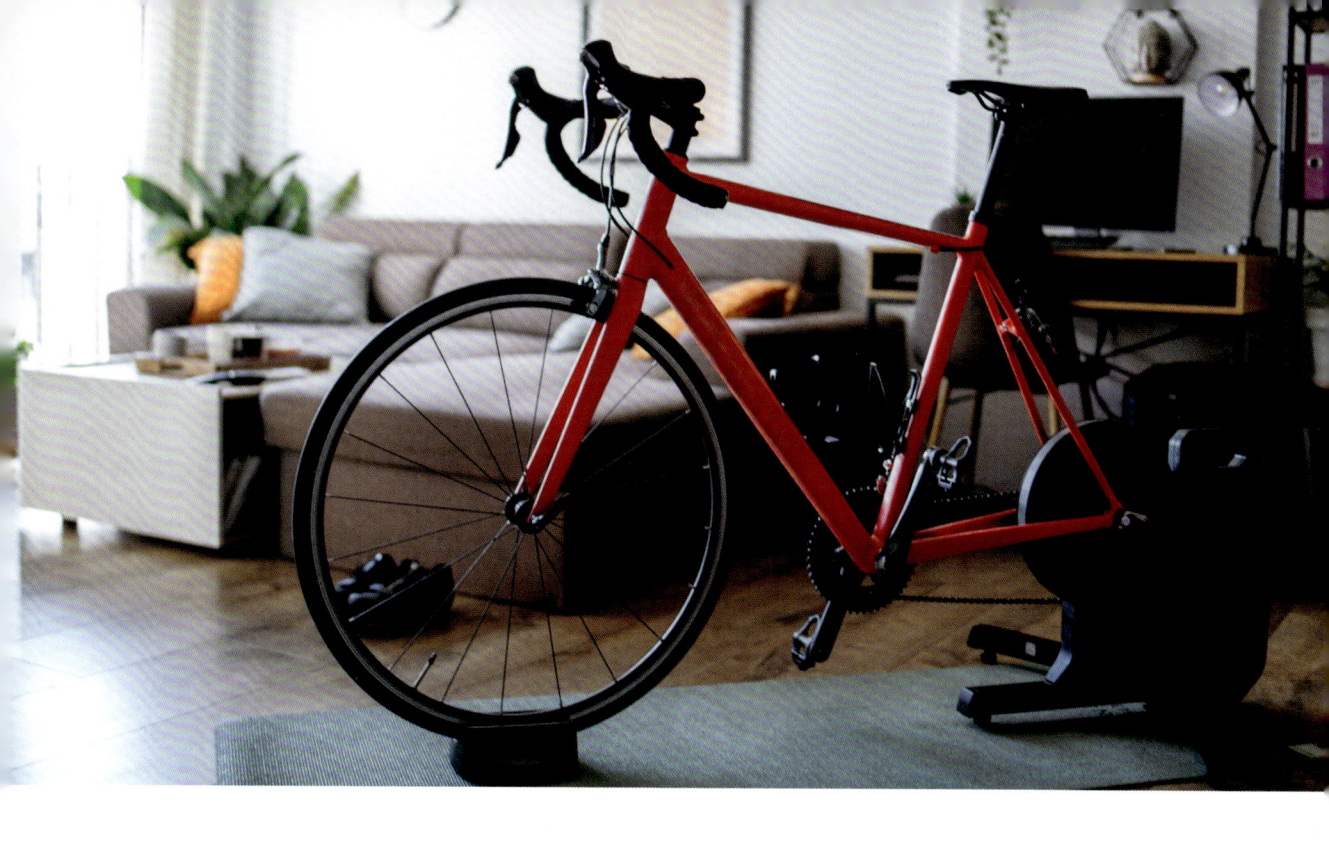

Over–unders
These are sometimes called lactate clearance intervals, because they aim to increase your body's efficiency at clearing lactate. They require you to ride above your FTP in order to create lactate, and then ride under your FTP, allowing the lactate to be consumed and cleared, and then repeating the process. They vary in length, but an aim would be to ride a set of three or four at two minutes at 105 per cent of FTP followed by two minutes at 90 per cent of FTP.

Flying 40s
These are fun but hard work. They involve one-minute pushes of 40 seconds at a very hard pace (110 per cent of FTP) followed by 20 seconds of easy peddling recovery. Try to reach 10 repetitions, but beware that there is not enough time for full recovery, so the intensity will build. Make sure you are not overdoing it and be prepared to step down a little.

Sweet spot
These moderate- to hard-paced sessions are more about improving aerobic and muscular endurance than anaerobic levels. They are based on a theory that there is a certain level of exertion that maximises your efficiency on the bike and allows you to recover faster than from high-intensity intervals. The magic is supposed to happen between 88 per cent and 94 per cent of FTP (a speed at which you can still get a few words out, but not hold a long conversation). If you can, do anything over 10 minutes. Sweet spot is a good alternative for those who lack the time for base training's long, slower rides or who find them too boring, and to keep up the endurance level as you ramp up the anaerobic training.

Tech has revolutionised the indoor cycling experience and even a small investment in a smart trainer can be a real eye-opener.

Smart trainers

Tech has revolutionised the indoor cycling experience and even a small investment in a smart trainer can be a real eye-opener. The popular choice is to buy a smart turbo (available for direct-drive and wheel-on turbos), which incorporates a power meter and allows external control of the level of resistance on the bike. It is possible to purchase smart rollers or even a speed and cadence sensor to make a basic roller compatible with most bike apps. By interacting with training apps, the real magic begins to happen.

When you enjoy your indoor sessions and they are not just a chore, you are going to get so much more out of them. The range of apps available open up an enormous range of activities, from basic training to entering a virtual world akin to a video game. They tend to be good in a particular area: apps like TrainerRoad, Peloton or Wahoo are good for interval training, while Rouvy and Bkool use augmented reality to put your avatar in real-world scenarios so you can 'ride' routes around the world, including the velodrome. Zwift is the big name in the market, providing a bit of everything, and is especially good for social interaction – racing and chatting to other riders. Apps are downloadable on to a phone or computer and range from free to a hefty subscription. Most offer some kind of free trial, so you can test them out before committing to a subscription.

Smart bike modes

The ergometer mode (ERG) setting on smart trainers and cycling apps locks in a target wattage and automatically adjusts the resistance to maintain the specific power level, regardless of your cadence or speed.

The sim (simulation) mode enables a 'real-life' scenario as it imitates the climbs and hills of a real outdoor road or course by varying the resistance of the bike according to the terrain.

Me and my trainer

I started on rollers back in my schooldays and used them more and more as I got into the sport. It was time-efficient and saved a whole lot of effort cleaning my bike. Indoor training was an important part of developing speed, but man it was boring and so uncomfortable just sitting there. I can cycle outside for six hours with no data and not get bored, but there's no way I could do that on an indoor trainer.

In my 20s, as a pro I had early access to power cranks and heart meters. That was a game-changer. It became more entertaining as you had various metrics – power, heart rate, cadence – to juggle as you rode. It was a game in itself. Now I love it. Zwift has made the whole thing fun. If I'm short of time, I do a one-hour ERG session. Other times, I warm up and see how I feel and whether I want to race or join a club ride. Often, I sit in the bunch just to watch what's going on. At my age, the trainer is by far the most productive way of maintaining fitness.

Fun time

Like a video game, many of the apps can easily become addictive. Zwift, for example, organises group rides, workouts and even races according to your FTP (for which it also provides tests, as do some other apps). The rides don't replicate real-life scenarios, but are set in an imaginary world called Watopia, which has 50 levels, each unlocking new routes – you need to be a level 6 to take on the Alpe Du Zwift, their version of the legendary Alpe d'Huez climb.

The popularity of the app is its key. If you want to race, there will always be one starting sometime soon, as there are riders all around the world jumping on. It's not quite like real racing, but there's enough of a similarity to get the adrenalin flowing with the ability to ride in groups, take advantage of the slipstream and launch an escape.

And whereas indoor training was once a solo endeavour, you need never be alone on a ride. You are able to send messages or even chat to individuals or groups. There are also plenty of clubs organising their own schedules of workouts, rides and races . . . check out the Chris Hoy rides!

RACING

Ed Clancy

For many – whatever their age – competitive cycling is the end game. Pitting yourself against others or even the clock can be daunting, but it is often the most exhilarating and exciting experience you can have on a bike.

Riders over 40 are welcomed at clubs and British Cycling events, but they are also specifically catered for at some clubs and by British Masters Cycle Racing (BMCR). The BMCR offer a year-round programme of road, circuit, track and gravel races for men and women. They have distinct age bands, but welcome all abilities, and novice and less-confident riders can compete in bands higher than their actual age group.

My world was the track, but I love road racing – watching and taking part in it. I truly believe it's the best sport in the world. It's so multidimensional. You ride as an individual, but also as part of a team, as a member of an ever-evolving and moving bunch, and in ad hoc collaborations that can disappear as quickly as they were formed.

Racing is exhilarating and great fun, but it isn't something to do on a whim. If you are not physically ready you will find yourself going backwards off the tail of the race pretty quickly and even be timed out. If you are not comfortable riding in a bunch, you may be a danger to yourself and others. Use club runs to practise and to gauge how ready you are. If you are not quite ready for a race, time trials are a good option. You don't have to worry about other riders or tactics; it is simply you against the track, usually over 16km (10 miles) or 40km (25 miles).

Racing takes some preparation and will take up the whole of a day. Entering a race doesn't mean you have to be intent on winning or even finishing among the top riders. Some cyclists race as part of their training and others just enjoy riding in the bunch without necessarily being competitive.

Of the general road races available, club bunch races are the most sociable, fun and low key; an Australian Pursuit Race (APR) is a handicap race where small groups of riders start at different times depending on ability; criteriums (or crits) are the shortest road races, but often the most technical; while British Cycling has four categories (not including the elite) with the fourth category being the entry level and moving up a level when the required points are gained from races in a season.

Racing is exhilarating and great fun, but it isn't something to do on a whim. If you are not physically ready you will find yourself going backwards.

The criterium is an all-action cycling race fought out on a short, closed circuit, usually in towns or cities, and usually lasting an hour. There are often over 100 riders, riding anything from 30 to 100 laps depending on the course. Fast and furious, they feature tight turns, short climbs and sometimes a sprint over cobblestones. A frantic start is commonly followed by frequent changes in pace with the race culminating in a sprint at breakneck speed. Crits suit technically adept riders who are able to recover quickly from short, high-intensity bursts.

Preparation is absolutely vital to even participating in a race. You need to have trained to a suitable level and, for British Cycling events, to have ridden in club bunch rides. You will need to have applied for the necessary licence (and insurance) to ride and completed the entry form in advance. Mark the race day in the diary and give yourself the best possible chance by timing your training, remembering to ease off in the days before the race. Getting the right amount of sleep and ensuring you consume enough protein, carbs and nutrients, and are well-hydrated, is critical.

Your bike should be immaculate; if it looks good, you'll feel good. Check everything and ensure that it is ready to ride. You will just be wasting time and money if your chain link breaks or the tyre blows out. If you are not confident about doing the maintenance yourself then take it to a bike shop to be serviced before the event.

This is the time to check the race course. If it is local, do a recce and ride it at least once to familiarise yourself with the route; if that isn't possible, check a map and utilise Google Maps and Street View. On the day before the race, give your bike another check-over and pack your clothes and plenty of gels, food and drinks. Take clothing for any eventuality. I make a 'rider' on the floor so I can see everything I've got. If I'm travelling to the start I pack it in order from the bottom to the top so I know where everything is. Always check and double-check you have your shoes. At a race, someone will have a spare of most things – socks, shorts, jerseys – that you can borrow. Except shoes. Without them, you can just turn around and go home.

On the day, I'll always turn up a couple of hours before the start. Everything takes longer than you think, from parking to signing in; even pinning on your numbers can take five or more minutes. Remember to consume any pre-race food or drink, check your bike and begin your warm-up 30 minutes before the start. On the

FULL GAS FOREVER

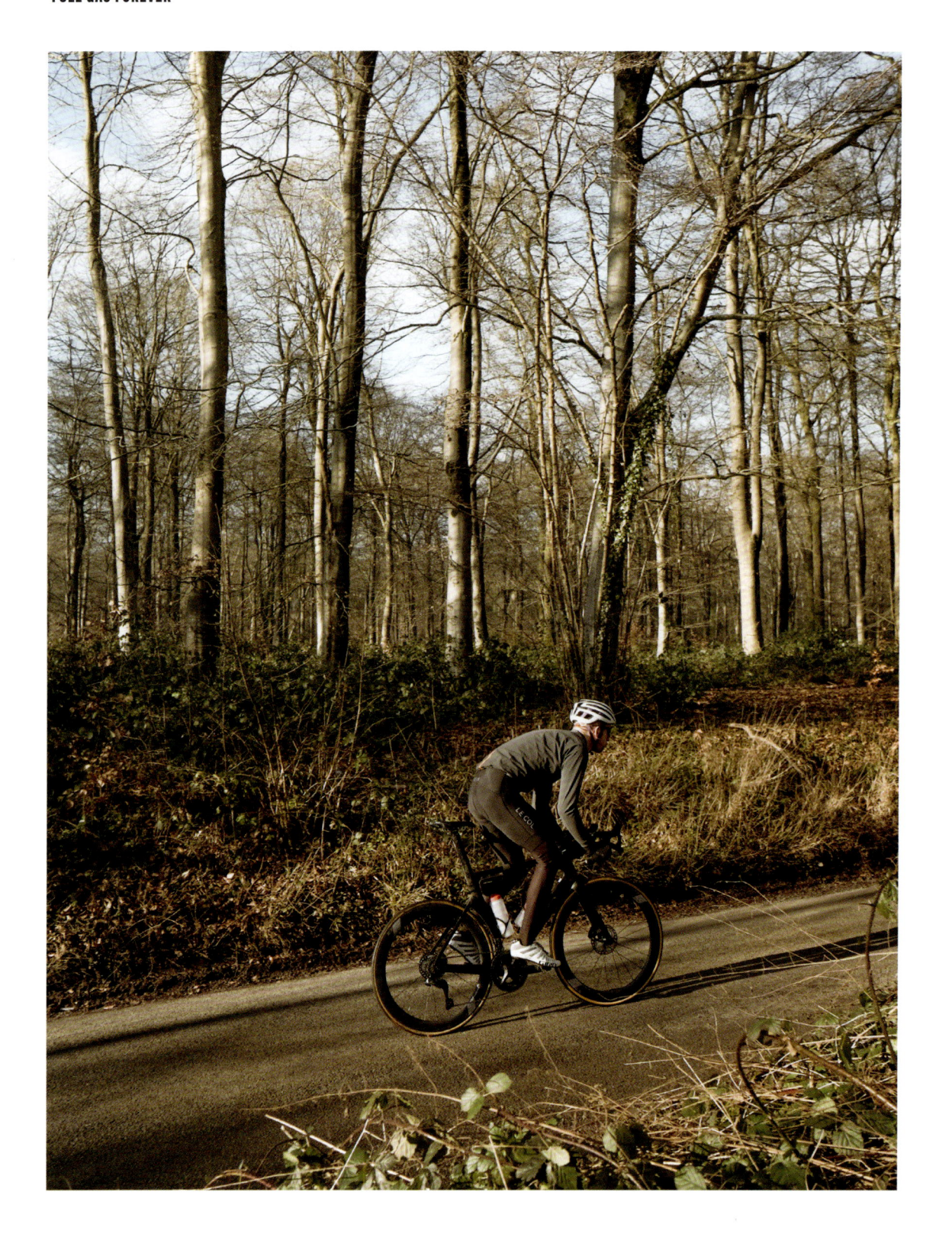

track we would have a 20-minute warm-up: five minutes to get settled and then progressively ramping up minute to minute from zone 3 to around FTP until we began to sweat. Then we'd just stay warm until the start. The exception can be on a criterium where if you are to be competitive any warm-up might have to be shortened in order to get a good starting position.

Limit your expectations for your first race. Some say 'staying upright' is a reasonable ambition. The pace will be much more furious than you will be used to and other riders will be less concerned with the niceties of club rides. Use it as a learning experience. Talk to people, get comfortable in the bunch, cover your brakes constantly and ride safely. Watch three or four riders ahead to spot obstacles or changes in speed, learn the etiquette and prepare to be yelled at. If you come last, so be it.

My first road race was as a 17-year-old. After 5km (3 miles) there was a big crash and I came out of it with a bent wheel. It was a scarring performance as I didn't have the money for a new wheel. For a while, I only rode in time trials. The moral of the story: only race if you accept that there is a chance you will crash and can bear the financial or physical damage.

Begin by using your energy wisely: don't attack; just follow. Stay in the front part of the bunch if you have the fitness and are comfortable, and remain constantly aware of what is going on around you. From your pre-race recce, be prepared for any hills, tricky sections, tight corners or open landscape where crosswinds could be an issue. If there is a steep climb, be aware that you might rapidly slide back down the bunch as better climbers go past you. In the approach, try to get yourself as far to the front as you can to ensure you don't end up losing touch at the back.

> **Only race if you accept that there is a chance you will crash and can bear the financial or physical damage.**

Tail-gunning

If you are new to racing, tail-gunning is a way of developing your confidence as a racer. In fact, depending on your ability, it may be the only option open to you. Position yourself at the back of the bunch and hang on to the group as best you can. Let people slot in front of you so you don't progress through the group. You can watch the race unfold without having to fight for position and you can keep a steady pace without having to slow down at corners and pinch points. Later in the race, if it opens out and you feel good, you might then begin to think about moving up. Tail-gunning can even be used as a tactic if the race has fewer than 40 entrants and is on flat, wide roads. It's not so effective if the route gets twisty and technical or has loads of riders (that said, Steve Cummings managed it regularly in the Tour de France!).

Reading the race is everything. Zwift and other apps are fun and progressing rapidly, but are still far from replicating real race experience. Racing can be like chess on wheels – not only guessing other riders' tactics and strategies, but assessing their fatigue levels and stamina. Try to understand how different scenarios can play out, what is going on with other riders' moves and how you can pre-empt or counter them. You can learn so much from YouTube videos or professional races on TV, but going out and racing is the only real place you will learn racing.

The 'concertina effect' (also called the 'accordion effect') is punishing for anyone at the rear of the race. It occurs when the bunch goes from a wide to a narrow road. From riding 10-abreast, riders are suddenly funnelled down to a road that is wide enough for four at a pinch. Apart from the first dozen riders, everyone else is forced to slow down, in increasing amounts back through the bunch with those towards the back even having to stop completely. It is a phenomenon that also happens at tight corners and where a number occur on one route it can have a significant effect on the race.

In any race, whether you are part of a team, are riding with some mates or have entered as an individual, you are never alone on the course. Allegiances and alliances are a crucial element of cycle racing. Try to get along with everyone and help out where you can. There's time for chatting along the way and you have at least one thing in common. This is the person who you might rely on to work with to bridge back to the bunch, to close down an escape or to help engineer your own breakaway. If you choose to upset someone – tagging on the back of the chain and not taking your turn, riding on someone's wheel for ages before going past them or getting physical in the final sprint – make sure it's worth it. Cyclists have long memories.

The last 3km (1.8 miles) is where the race is often won or lost. If you are at the front and have paced yourself right, you are in with a chance of finishing among the top riders. This is the part of the race you should have committed to memory. Where are the corners? How steep are the hills? Is the finish on a hilltop or at the end of a long straight? Every finish is different, but the basics remain the same. Make sure you are in the right gear, watch any riders around you like a hawk, be aware of your own strengths and weaknesses – can you sprint more effectively over a shorter or longer distance? – and either seize an opportunity that arises or wait to choose your moment to make your move. That might need patience; some say only put your nose in the wind once – when you cross the line.

Finishing a race can be emotional and physically draining, but stick to your post-race routine. Warm down properly, get warm clothes on if it is a cold day and consume any recovery food or drink you have brought – even if it is the last thing you fancy at that moment. While it is fresh in your mind, take a few moments to assess the race: what you did well, mistakes you made and lessons you learned. Remember that you learn more from your failings than your successes.

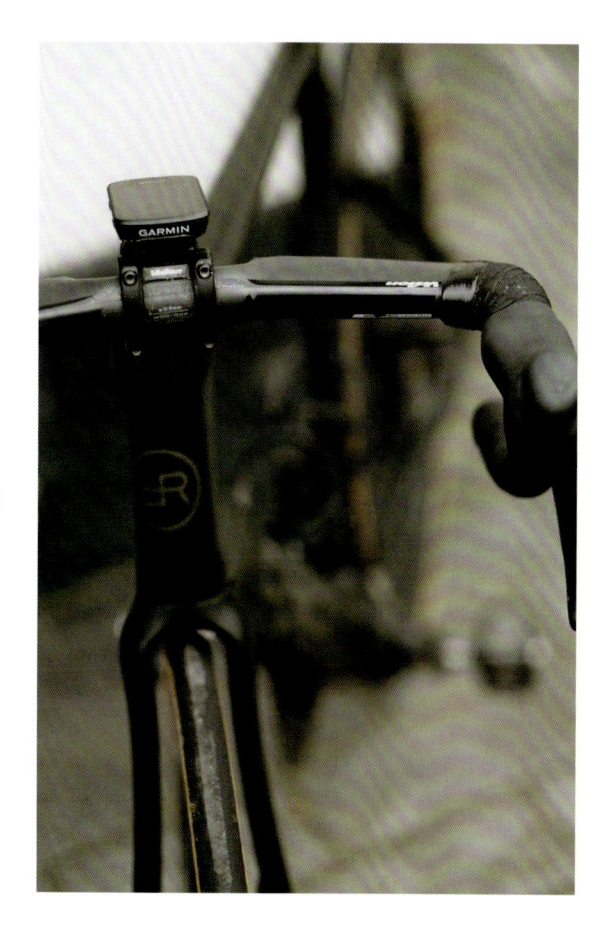

Remember that you learn more from your failings than your successes.

Be more like Cav

A huge part of Mark Cavendish's success as a cyclist was his racing intelligence. No one understood a race like him. From an early age he was obsessed with racing and tactics, especially in bunch sprints. When he debriefed a race it was incredible. He knew who was there and what they were doing, like he saw the whole thing in slow motion. It was a skill that enabled him to think in an instant and make the right decision.

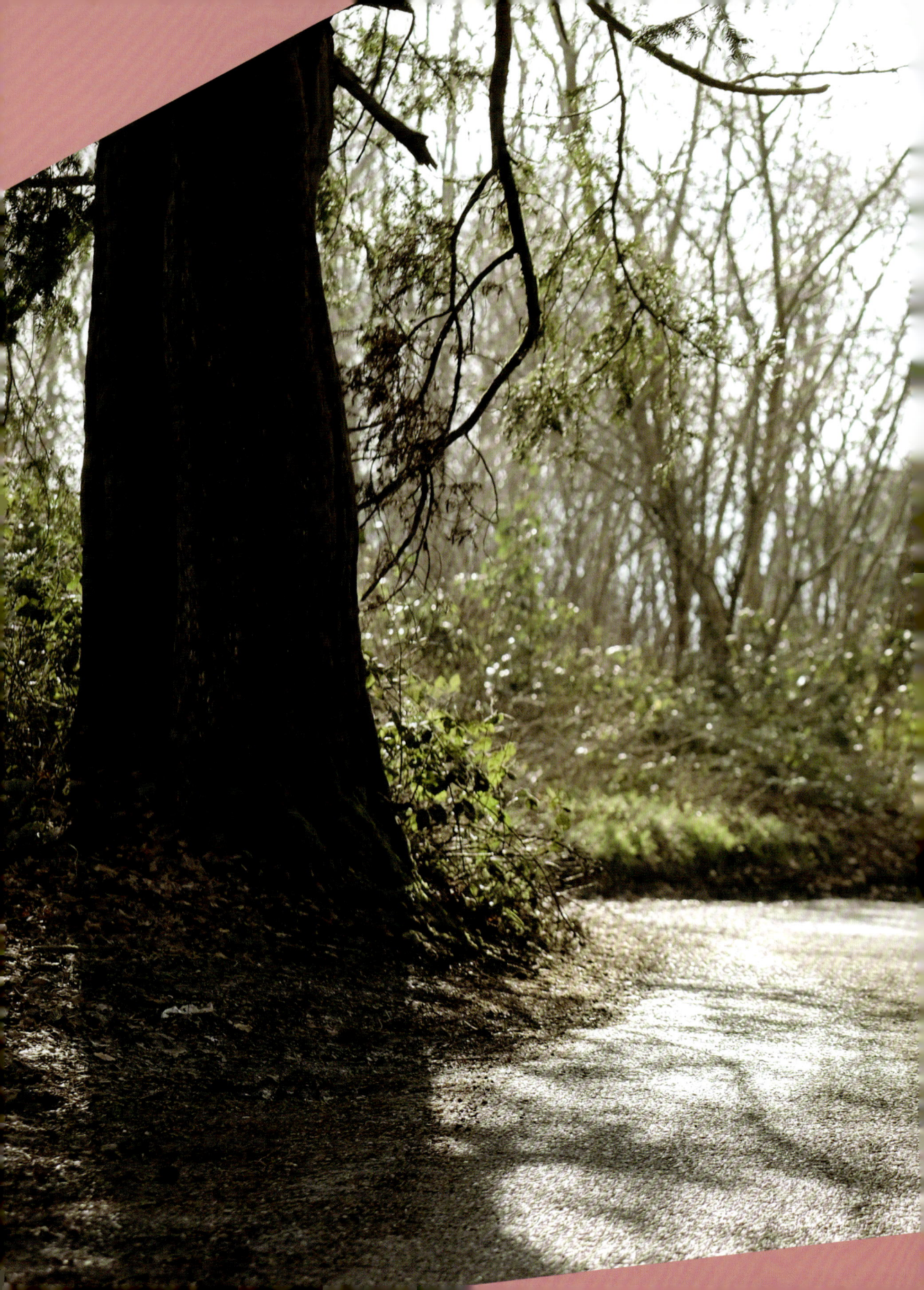

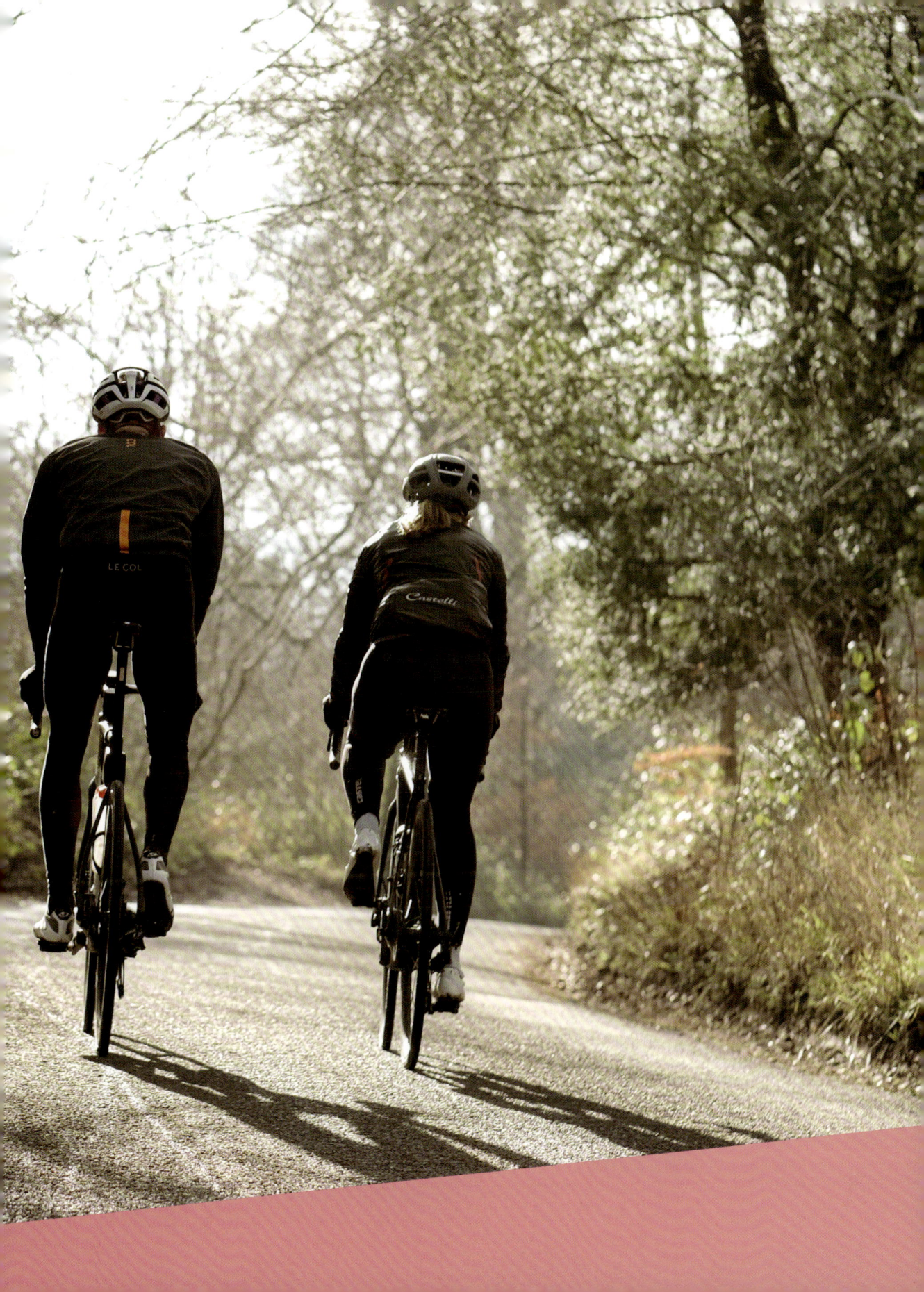

SPORTIVES, GRAN FONDO'S AND ÉTAPES

Ed Clancy

Now almost the natural habitat of the mature cyclist, mass-participation rides are simple to enter, but not always so easy to finish.

If you think you are ploughing a lone furrow as a 40-, 50- or 60-year old cyclist then you haven't been on a mass-participation ride – a sportive, gran fondo or Étape du Tour – where older riders are often in the majority. The last decade or more has seen a proliferation of these organised rides in the UK and overseas, and they are particularly targeted at reasonably fit cyclists looking for a different terrain or experience. Though tremendous fun, these mass-participation rides represent a serious endeavour. They can be physically and technically challenging, and provide great motivation for training and a chance to assess your fitness and ability.

The categories of the rides are blurred. Some use the Italian term 'gran fondo', which translates as 'big ride', while in the UK and France 'sportive' is generally used for similar kinds of rides. These are all one-day, long-distance events. They vary in length, but tend to be over 100km (62 miles) with shorter options sometimes available, and are ridden over a circuit or between specific points with support such as feeding stations or mechanical assistance provided. Organisers find it increasingly difficult to close roads to other traffic, so in most cases expect well-signed routes marshalled by volunteers and police.

What can vary from ride to ride is the start. There is the traditional gran fondo mass start where anything up to 3000 riders assemble at the start line, while sportives often use staggered starts of more manageable numbers where you turn up in a time slot with a chip to record your time or wait in pre-designated starting 'pens' according to the time in which you expect to complete the ride.

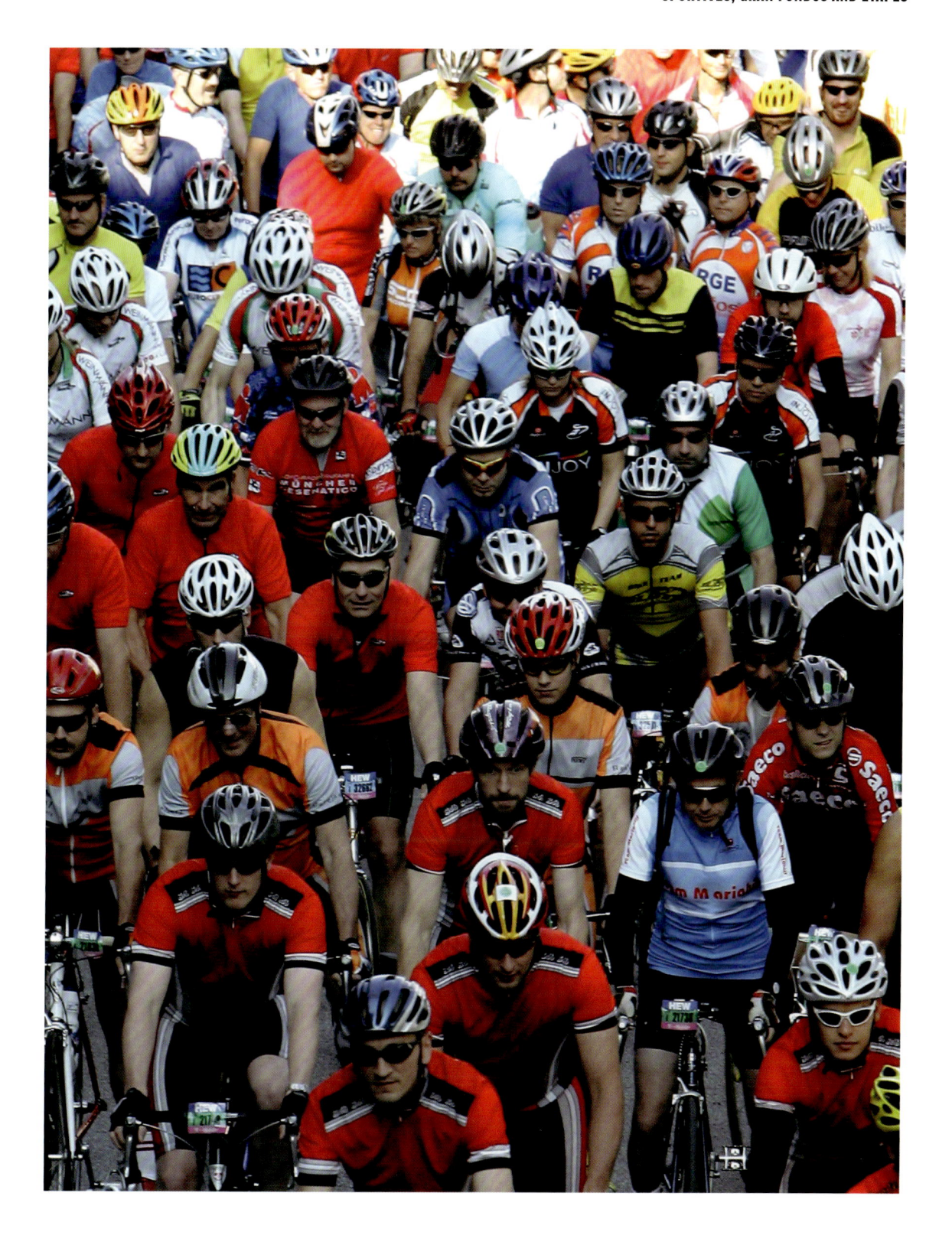

SPORTIVES, GRAN FONDOS AND ÉTAPES

FULL GAS FOREVER

Training for a sportive or similar is the same as for any ride: build up your base fitness, keep your training progressive and ease off in the week before the event.

The important thing to understand is that none of these rides (with the exception of some Italian grand fondos) are races. Some might give that impression with published individual times, prizes, kitted-up riders eager to start at the front and some jostling for position before a major climb, but it's a choice: compete or complete – and most choose the latter. Some will ride it more as a time trial with their own objective in mind, while a great many will just be aiming to finish. Staying within the regular time checks along the route can often be testing enough.

Training

Training for a sportive or similar is the same as for any ride: build up your base fitness, keep your training progressive and ease off in the week before the event. Train with the specific event in mind. How long is it and what kind of time cut-offs are you looking at? As a rule of thumb you will be expected to average at least 14km/h (9mph). In contrast to racing, a sportive or gran fondo is about stamina, not speed.

You will be on the road for six hours or more and will need to maintain a steady pace, so ensure your training programme includes some long rides to see how you cope and how your fuelling strategy works. Make sure you feel as comfortable as you can. If your neck or your butt feels sore after a three-hour ride, just imagine how it is going to feel after double that. Check or experiment with your bike set-up and put in the hours on the saddle on training rides.

Ride the full distance of the planned event or 80–90 per cent of it at least once to give you an idea of how to pace yourself and what kind of time to aim for. You may well find you fare better than expected as adrenaline, motivation, drafting and the support of others around you can really help you on the day. Most popular routes also feature some serious climbing, which can come as a shock if you are just used to rolling hills. If you don't want to join those pushing your bike up the switchbacks it might be a good idea to seek out the nearest challenging ascent to get some practice in pacing yourself on a climb, riding a low cadence and getting out of the saddle.

Finally, a number of these rides will involve cycling at altitude. People's responses to high-elevation riding vary considerably. There is little you can do in advance (unless you have time to fully acclimatise) except to make sure you are aware that the decreased availability of oxygen can impact performance. You will likely find it more physically and nutritionally demanding, so adapt your training, and your food and liquid intake, accordingly.

Preparation

There's no point in spending good money, taking time off work and training hard if you are not prepared, and in the right state of mind, for an event. Much of the advice for preparation for a race is applicable here, too. Get your bike checked over and your clothes, bike and other bits and pieces ready in plenty of time. If you are not going on a package, then you will need to make sure you have your flight (with bike) booked and hotel accommodation reserved (they can get booked up early). Flying with your bike is remarkably easy with a suitable bike box or bag for the flight, but put your shoes and pedals in your cabin luggage – that way, if your luggage goes missing (it happens!) you can get everything else at the event.

Get there in plenty of time. Many riders make a mini-break of it, travelling with friends, partners or family. It gives you time to relax, to have a pre-ride or two and, hopefully, you will get some support on the big climb. On the day, you won't need a lot. Some organisers insist on you taking a rain cape, and a pump and spare tube are recommended. Any other mechanical issues should just entail a short wait for one of the help cars to arrive and sort it for you. Carry a few gels just in case and a couple of full 750ml (25fl oz) bidons, but nearly all these events are well catered. The feed stations are numerous and offer a great choice of energy drinks, snacks and bars, sandwiches and pasta.

Most of the events are amazingly well organised. You will probably receive a GPS map download that not only shows the route in detail, but also provides valuable information on climbs, descents and other potentially tricky points along the route. It also marks the time limit at each of the cut-off points. It's worth noting if you think that could be an issue.

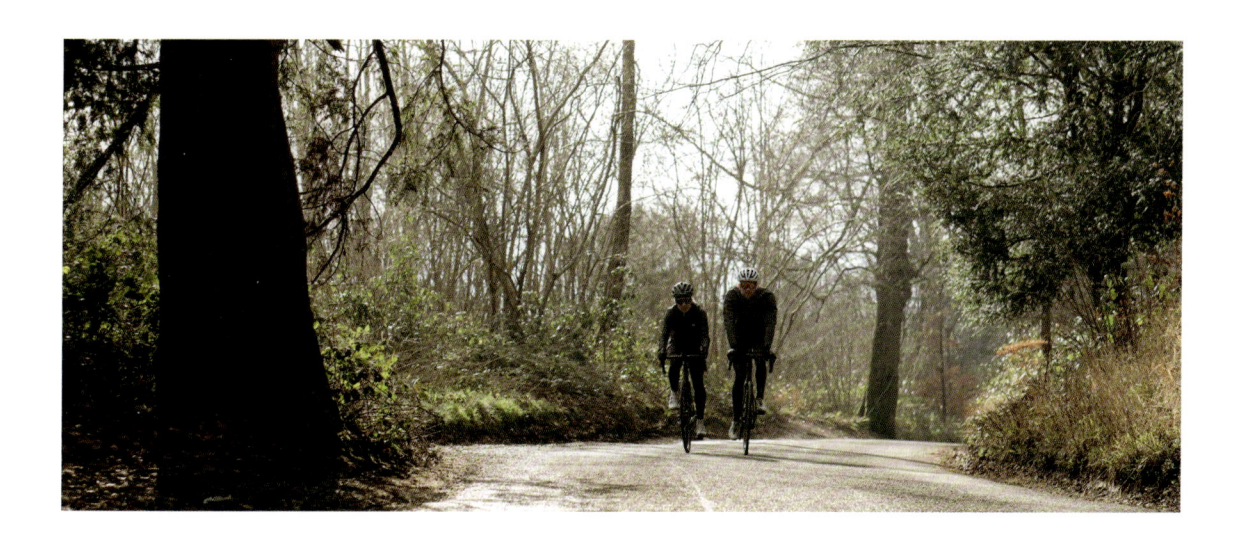

FULL GAS FOREVER

Preparation is everything, as the following stories demonstrate! Because of work commitments I flew out late to an étape that involved riding the course of the penultimate day of the Tour de France. I got to the hotel the night before, too late to get a decent meal, and got up at 5.00 a.m. as we were in the first starting pen. I had something for breakfast, but didn't feel like much, and then found I had a squidgy tyre, but I had forgotten my pump so I had to borrow one on the start line. I was sleep-deprived and under-fuelled, had a slow in my back tyre and still had to ride 130km (80 miles) negotiating steep climbs on bad roads at altitude. I was knackered from start to finish and though it was nice riding with friends, I could have got so much more from the day.

Compare that to my experience at the Gran Fondo Alberto Contador on the Costa Blanca. I flew out 48 hours before it began, which gave me time to have a short ride and check my bike was fine, and chill out with my pals. We looked at the route profile and put a loose strategy together. On the day, I was out in the front group with Ian Bibby, Alex Dowsett, Jesse Yates and others, just pushing it a little and having such a great time.

On the ride

When you arrive at the event, there is a totally different vibe to a race. This is more like a festival with stalls, music, speakers and food stands. It is totally relaxed and friendly. Get a few cyclists together and some are bound to race, but after the first proper climb it will be obvious who are the competitors and who are the completers. The vast majority fall into the completers category. They are there to have a good time and finish the course.

If you're one of the many completers, these tips will apply:

- For a beginner, a crowded start can be fraught. If you feel anxious then position yourself to the rear of the pack before the ride begins.
- Don't let the adrenaline get to you. The first few kilometres can be frenetic. Let the others go, and do your own thing.
- Watch out for other riders. Even those who look the part may not share your technical ability.
- Keep fuelled. If you miss out on a feed station there may not be another for a couple of hours.
- Stay hydrated. You might well be cycling in hotter or more humid conditions than you are used to and need to take on more water than usual.
- Go careful on the descents. It's tempting to think you can make up time, but they can be dangerous, so take it easy.
- Drafting isn't cheating. Take someone's wheel for a while; you can always offer to take a turn at the front.
- Pace yourself, ride within your limits and savour that feeling when you cross the finish line.

Sportive selection

There are so many mass-participation rides available that you are spoilt for choice at every level. If you are looking to push yourself they are a great way to ride as hard as you can with no worries about directions, food or technical support – but of course, it all comes at a price. The bigger rides can be really popular, so it's worth getting organised and registering as far in advance as possible or looking for one of the charity fund-raising places available.

You can find some really testing sportives without even leaving the UK. The biggest, RideLondon, was one of the few closed-road events in the country. It took a hiatus in 2025, but hopefully will be back in 2026. The Dragon Ride offers four routes from 100km (60 miles) to 350km (220 miles) across the mountains of mid-Wales, including the 1.5km (1 mile)-long Devil's Staircase with its 25 per cent gradients. One of my favourite sportives is the one they call 'the Daddy', the Fred Whitton Challenge. It takes you on a 180km (112 mile) route over the mountains of the Lake District and is deemed the toughest one-day event in Britain. There are plenty of gravel options too, with their unique vibe. They range from the challenging Dirty Reiver in Kielder Forest near the Scottish Borders to Grinduro in South Wales, which is part festival and part race.

If you are willing to venture further there are étapes that follow the route of stages of the Tour de France or the classics, so you, too, can brave the cobbles of the Tour of Flanders or Paris–Roubaix. The original, La Marmotte, which includes the climbs of Galibier and Alpe d'Huez, sells out its 7000 places in no time. On mainland Europe you are more likely to find closed-road routes: Mallorca has become a haven for Northern European cyclists and Mallorca 312 offers a gruelling 300km (186 miles) or more tour of the island with 5000m (16,400ft) of climbing. In the home of the gran fondo – Italy – you will find events such as the Maratona dles Dolomites and La Stelvio Santini Granfondo, which transverses the Stelvio Pass, one of the highest paved mountain passes in Europe.

If you are willing to venture further there are tapes that follow the route of stages of the Tour de France or the classics, so you, too, can brave the cobbles of the Tour of Flanders or Paris–Roubaix.

EPILOGUE, ED CLANCY

IN MANY WAYS WE ARE the luckiest generation. A combination of science, technology and fitness advances have given us an unequalled opportunity to carry on and improve our cycling right into our senior years. There is absolutely nothing stopping us getting on a bike for the first time as a mature person and enjoying the excitement of speed on two wheels or taking our cycling to levels our younger selves never had the opportunity, time or inclination to reach.

We hope this book has been both a guide and a source of encouragement and self-belief to improving as a cyclist. We want you to feel that improving your performance in your middle age or beyond is, if not easy, a pretty straightforward process. Sure, age works against you in some respects, but when didn't it? Careers, childcare, finance, a frantic lifestyle . . . life always throws up obstacles. Hopefully, we have shown that any age-related constraints to meeting your cycling ambitions are either in the mind or fairly simply overcome with some sensible guidelines and training.

Potential is not something that diminishes with age. Willpower does not disappear as the wrinkles and first grey hairs appear, and dreams are not the sole property of youth. Being part of a speeding chain gang, going on a daring escape, reaching a mountain-top climb or just finishing that century ride can be as thrilling at 48 as it was at 18. Go on, get out there. . . . You know you can do it.

Potential is not something that diminishes with age. Willpower does not disappear as the wrinkles and first grey hairs appear and dreams are not the sole property of youth.

EPILOGUE

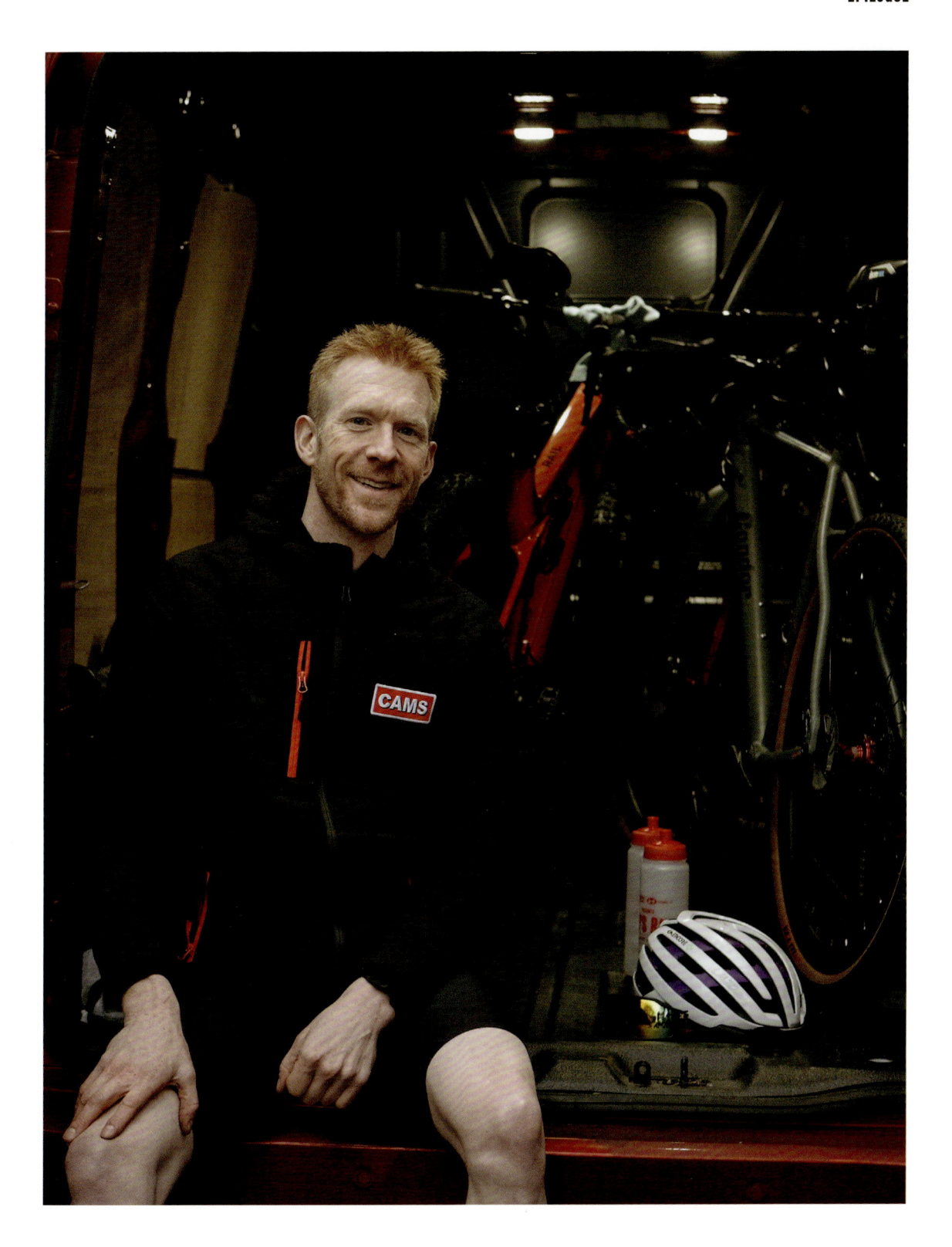

FULL GAS FOREVER

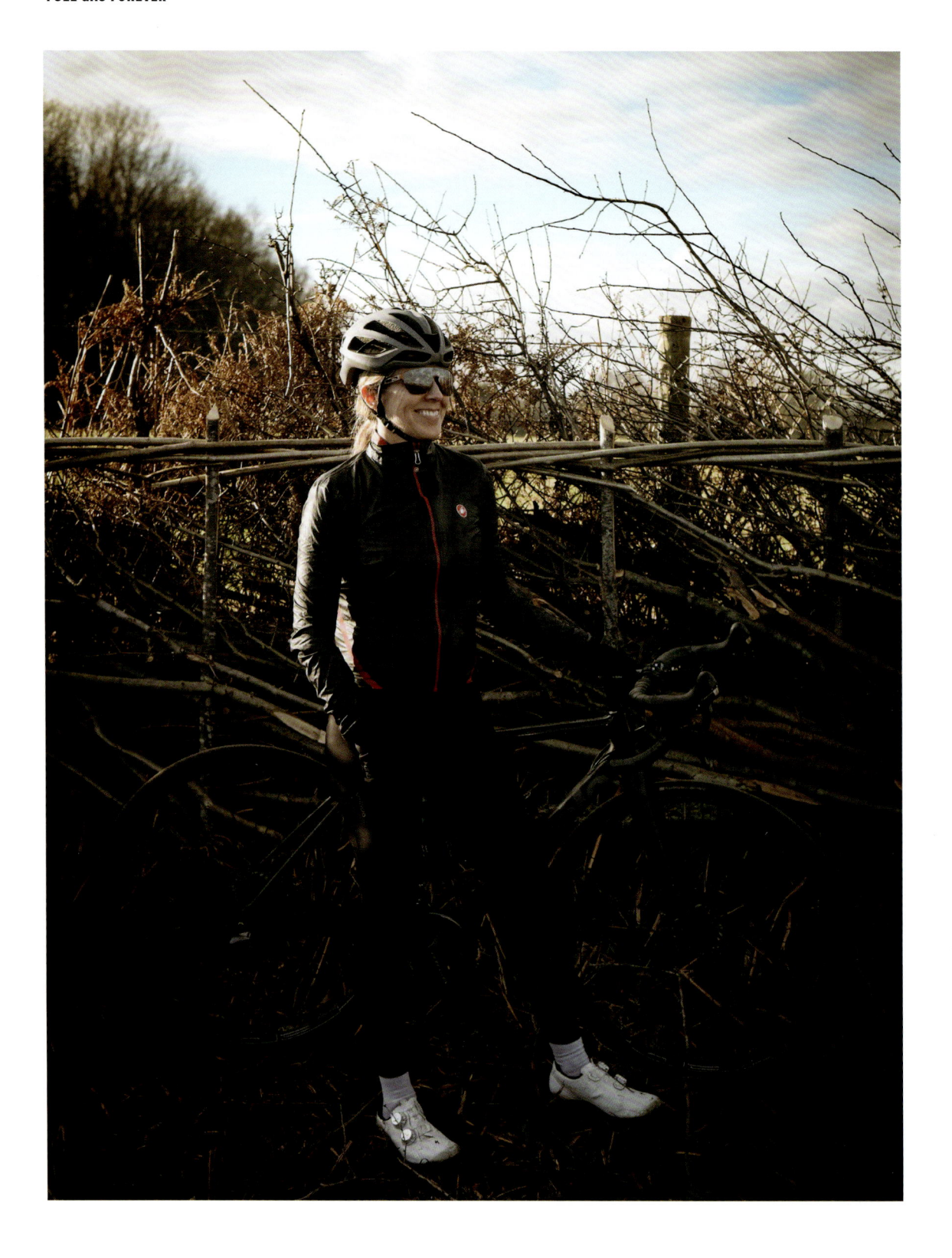

EPILOGUE, LEXIE WILLIAMSON

STUDIES HAVE SHOWN THAT VO$_2$ max is one of the strongest predictors of longevity, along with leg strength, exercise levels and muscle mass. Not to be smug, but for us serious older cyclists, having the oxygen absorption prowess of a 20-year-old and thighs of steel come as standard. As does an exercise addiction.

So, the signs are already there then for a long life filled with many happy hours in the saddle.

But are we content with merely spinning the legs and accepting a slow downward slide into mediocrity? Or do we want to continue to sweat and suffer through midlife and beyond, bagging PRs, cups and summits?

Most of us want the latter and rightly so. Cycling is one of the few sports where you can continue to push your body to peak performance in your 40s, 50s and 60s.

We are arguably the first few generations to test these perceived age limitations and are riding long after previous generations had hung up their bib shorts.

But there is always more to learn and I sincerely hope that this book has provided a few nuggets that can be incorporated into your future training – either from the legend that is three-times Olympic gold medallist Mr Clancy, who mines his vast experience of all things training, or the experts I consulted on nutrition, sleep, hormones and more.

I have certainly learned a few things. As a perimenopausal, vegetarian rider I was seriously under-consuming protein so I am now doubling up on eggs and beans. I am also versed in the art of the nappuccino, can conduct a DIY sweat test and have finally picked up those weights after the evidence of its benefits for bone density, hormone depletion and more popped up chapter after chapter.

My favourite gain, however, from writing this book is discovering that high-intensity interval training releases not just dopamine but also the love hormone oxytocin. So, it's not a fleeting obsession; you really are in love with cycling.

Here's to many more epic years of fun and full gas.

REFERENCES

Chapter 1

'Some scientific research has also revealed there is a link between strong legs and a fit brain' UF Health, *Strong legs linked to brawny brain*, UF Health, 4/4/16 https://ufhealth.org/stories/2016/strong-legs-linked-to-brawny-brain

'Dr Kenneth Cooper, a pioneer of the use of aerobic exercise to maintain and improve health, is useful': Kenneth H Cooper, *Aerobics, M.Evans, 1968*

'scientists now believe that happens after the age of 60': P-15 Herman Pontzer et al, *Daily energy expenditure*, Science Journal, 13/8/2021, https://www.science.org/doi/10.1126/science.abe5017

'Older cyclists should pay greater heed to hydration as they have less body water': Andy Blow, *Does an endurance athlete's hydration needs change as they age?*, 220 Triathalon, 15/11/23, https://www.220triathlon.com/training/nutrition-training/does-an-endurance-athletes-hydration-needs-change-as-they-age

Chapter 9

'The limited research available suggests that fasted training is not advisable for women': Dr Stacy Sims, *Why women should never exercise on an empty stomach*, Unfiltered, 18/5/2024, https://unfilteredonline.com/dr-stacy-sims-why-women-should-never-exercise-on-an-empty-stomach

Chapter 11

'Hormonal fluctuations can also affect aerobic fitness': https://www.balance-menopause.com/menopause-library/fit-and-active-how-the-menopause-can-affect-you/

'Peri-menopausal and menopausal women should also bear in mind that these measurements': Dr Hussain, *Fit and active? How the menopause can affect you*,

Chapter 12

'There's also research demonstrating that as you get older your body becomes less efficient at producing those 'thirsty' signals': Andy Blow, *Does an endurance athlete's hydration needs change as they age?*, 220 Triathalon, 15/11/23, https://www.220triathlon.com/training/nutrition-training/does-an-endurance-athletes-hydration-needs-change-as-they-age

BIBLIOGRAPHY

Bean, Anita, *The Complete Guide to Sports Nutrition*, 9th edition, Bloomsbury, 2022

Cavell, Phill, *The Midlife Cyclist*, Bloomsbury, 2021

Murchison, Alan, *The Cycling Chef*, Bloomsbury, 2019

Williamson, Lexie, *Yoga for Cyclists*, 2nd edition, Bloomsbury, 2024

ACKNOWLEDGEMENTS

We would like to thank all the experts consulted for this book. They are Phil Cavell, Bianca Broadbent, Bryan McCullough, Graham Theobald, Emily Arrell, Jonathan Baker, Anita Bean and Alan Murchison.

Big shout also to our photographer Tony Blake, who produced the images on a crisp sunny morning in the Surrey Hills, and of course to the hardworking Bloomsbury duo Sarah Skipper and Matt Lowing who were always on hand to share their publishing expertise and guide us.

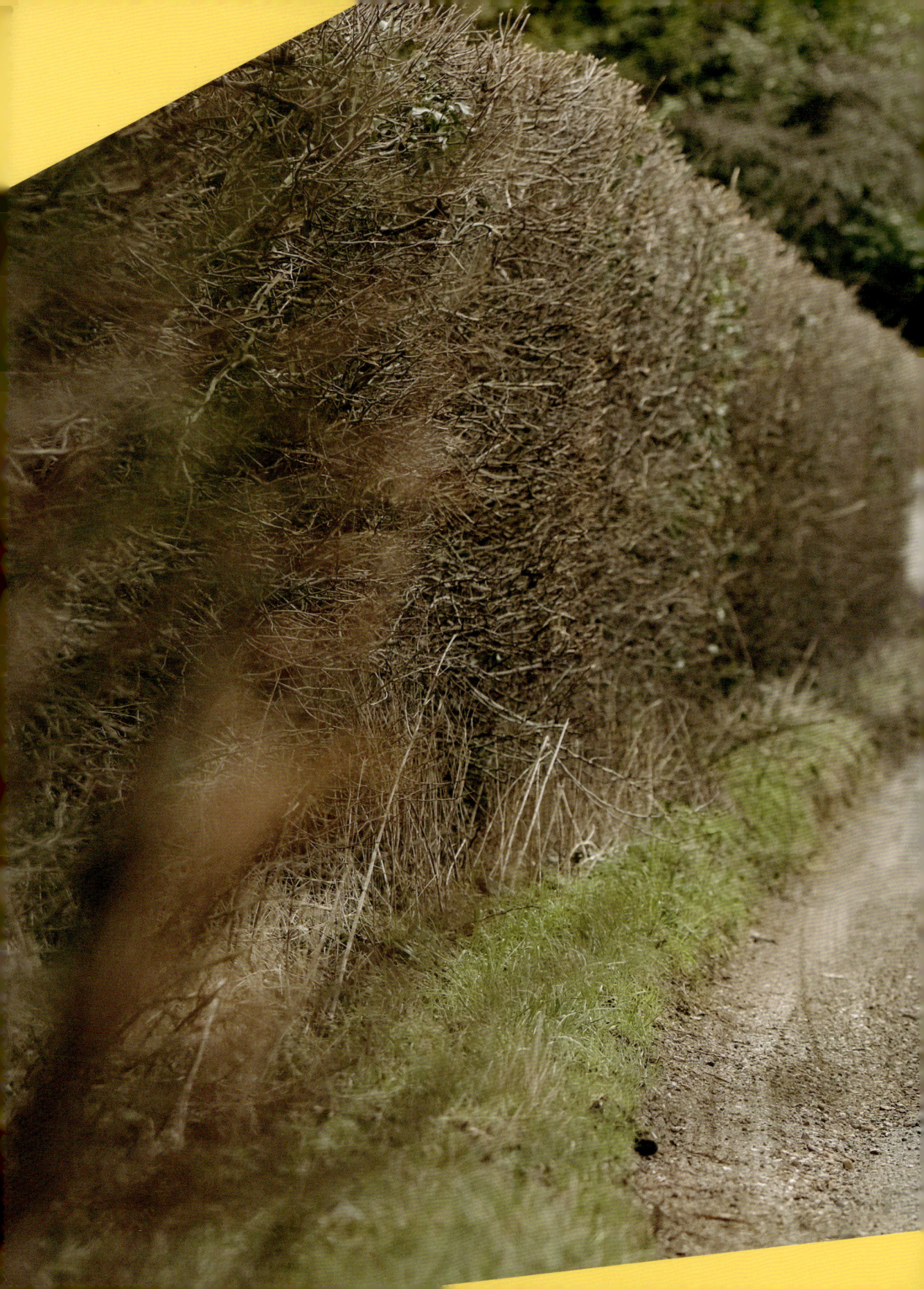

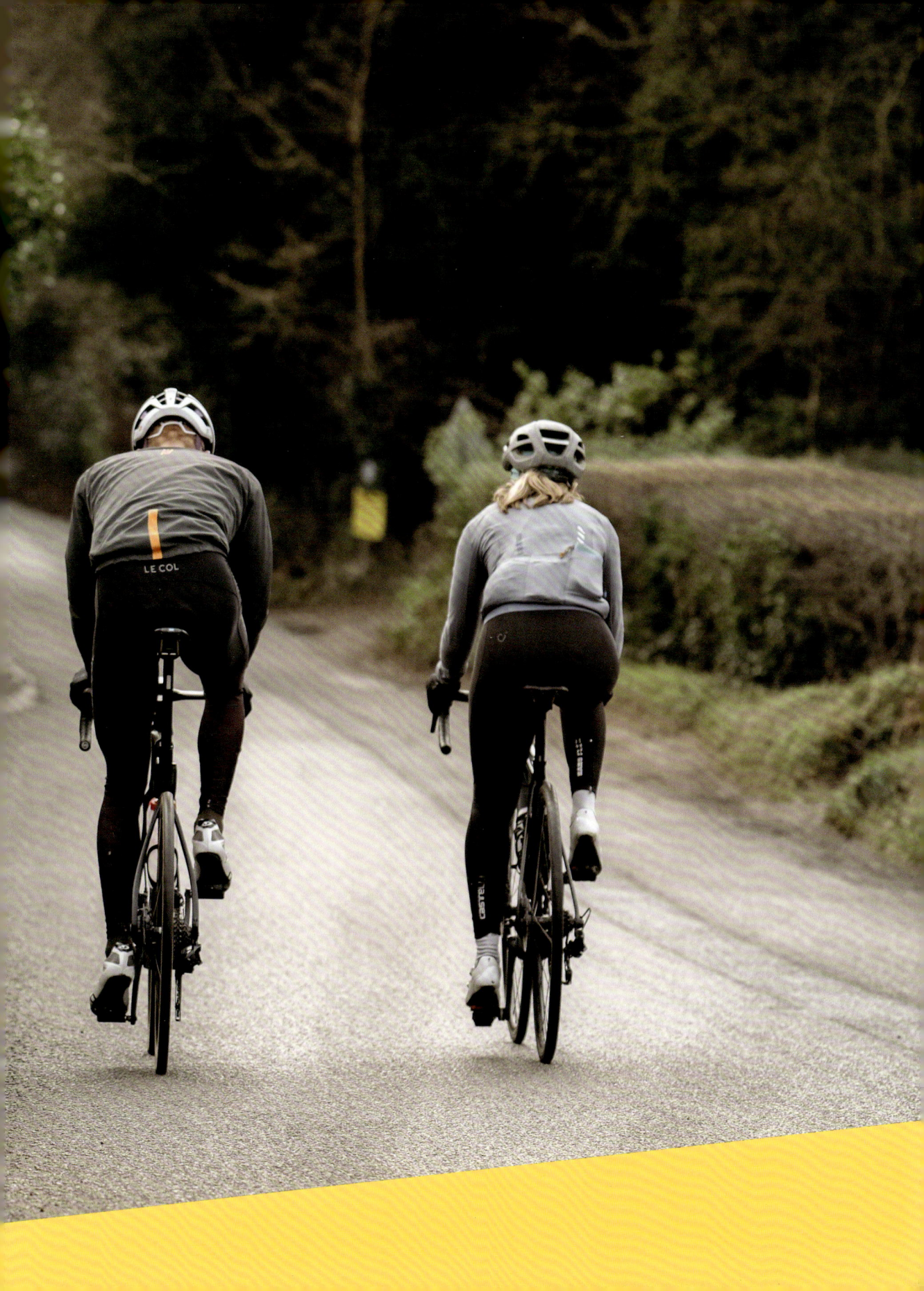

INDEX

A
aerobic base 13
aerodynamic drag/air resistance 56–61
apps 83, 94, 96, 167
Arrell, Emily 118–19

B
base training 93–4
Bean, Anita 128–9, 131
benefits 12–13
bent-leg windscreen wiper 47
bike fit *see* set up
bikes 18–25
bird dog 49
bodyweight squat 33
bodyweight strength training 29–36
Brailsford, Dave 86
brakes 18–19
braking 105
breathing exercises 143
bridges
   glute 35
   hamstring 35
   rolling 46
   single leg hamstring 45
British Masters Cycle Racing (BMCR) 168
Burt, Phil 59
buttock pain 80

C
cadence 102–5
caffeine 120–1, 140, 141
calcium 127
carbohydrates
   carbohydrate-fasted training 97
   and nutrition 128–9
Cavell, Phil 26, 27, 124, 149, 150
Cavendish, Mark 59, 173
chains, maintenance 24
cleats 59–60
clothing 61
coffee 120–1, 140, 141
confidence 89
Cooper, Kenneth 13

Coppi, Fausto 91
core, defined 43
core strength 14
   exercises 44–53
   high-performance chassis (HPC) 42–3
cornering 105, 107
cramps 119
cranks 60
cyclo-cross 156–7

D
delayed onset muscle soreness (DOMS) 27, 134–5
diet/nutrition 15, 17, 124–31
   and hormones 146–7, 150
   and recovery 133
   and sleep 140
drafting 107
dumbbell side bend 48

E
electric bikes 156

F
fatigue 135
feedback 89
figure-four 67
flexibility 15, 62–3
   exercises 64–73
floor swimmer 32
flying 40s 165
forearm plank 45
frames 24
Froome, Chris 59
functional threshold power (FTP) 96, 110, 165, 167

G
gears 24
gels 125
glute bridge 35
glycogen 138
goblet squat 37

gravel racing 157, 159
group riding 98
gyms 39

H
hamstring bridge 35
hamstring hang 68
hamstring strap stretch 68
hand release push-up 31
handlebars 21–3, 59
heart rate variability 137
helmets 61
Henderson, Neal 137
high-intensity interval training (HIIT) 14
high-performance chassis (HPC) 42–3
hills 98
hips
   flexors 71
   pain 78
hormones 146–51
Hoy, Chris 86
human growth hormone (HGH) 138, 149
hydration 17, 94, 116–21

I
indoor training 162–7
injuries 76–83, 91
interval training 109–10
   and hormones 151
iron supplements 127

K
kneeling hand release push-up 30
kneeling lat stretch 68
kneeling push-up plank 30
knees, injuries/pain 82–3

L
lactate threshold (LTHR) 109–10
lateral flexion 72
lateral leg lift 47
lateral leg swing 64
lateral squat 37

INDEX

legs, hairy 60
low lunge 67
lunges
  low 67
  reverse 34
  standing 70
  tipping 64
lying twist 51, 66

M

McCullough, Brian 80, 81, 83
maintenance, bike 25, 169
Marcora, Samuele 135
mass-participation rides 176–81
mental performance 84–91
  interval 109–10
  overtraining 14, 111
  polarisation and periodisation 110–11
mid-back loosener 65
motivation 84–6, 87–9
mountain biking 19, 20, 21, 24, 59, 152–6
Murchison, Alan 125, 129

N

napping 139, 140, 141
neck tension 81
90-degree long roller/wall stretch 71
90/90 leg swing 65
nutrition *see* diet/nutrition

O

oestrogen 148–9
off-road 152–9
Olympic training 108
omega-3 fatty acids 127
overtraining 14, 111, 134
over–unders 165
oxytocin 151

P

pain 15
  buttock 80
  hip 78
  knees 82–3
  lower back 79
  and mental performance 91
  neck 81
Panayiotou, Chris 27–9
parachute lift 45
pedalling 102–5
pedals 24
periodisation 110–11
Peters, Steve 7, 86, 87, 89
planks
  forearm 45
  forearm plank into plank 49
  side plank rotation 45
plateauing 111
polarisation 110–11
posture 15, 52–3, 164
power meters 96
programmes, training 113–15
progressive training 13, 97, 111
prone quad stretch 66
prone snow angel 53
protein 124, 126, 131, 149
  and recovery 133
puppy dog stretch 66

R

racing 168–73
rate of perceived exertion 96–7, 134
recovery 17, 132–7
  and hormones 150
  and hydration 121
  nutrition 128
relaxation exercises 143
repeated bout effect 135–6
resistance, air *see* aerodynamic drag/air resistance
resistance training 26, 27, 150
rest days 38, 90–1, 132
  nutrition 129
resting heart rate 136–7
reverse lunge 34
reverse tabletop 45
rolling bridge 46
Russian twist 48

S

sacrifice 34
saddles 19–20, 58–9
sarcopenia 27, 125
seated cat stretch 50
seated twist 72
set up 15, 57–8
  cleats 59–60
  cranks 60
  handlebars 59
  indoor trainers 164
  saddles 58–9
setbacks 90–1
side plank rotation 45
single leg hamstring bridge 36
skydiver 32
sleep 15, 138–41, 150
  exercises 142–3
  and recovery 133–4
slipstreams 107
smart trainers 166–7
sphinx crunch 46
spinal extension 73
spinal flexion 73
sportives 176–81
squats
  bodyweight 33
  goblet 37
  lateral 37
stability ball mountain climber 48
standing lunge 70
standing (or seated) fold 51
standing single arm row via a door frame 33
static mountain climber 50
static split squat 34
stiff leg deadlift 38
strap pec stretch 53
strength training 14, 26–8
  bodyweight 29–36
  exercises 29–39
stress 150
stretching *see* flexibility
success 89–90
supplements 127
sweating 116–17, 118, 119, 162–3
sweet spots 165

T

Tabata 164
tail-gunning 172–3
tapering 111, 113
technique 102–7
technology 14–15
　smart trainers 166–7
testosterone 146–8
Theobald, Graham 82, 83
30–30s 164
Thomas, Geraint 24, 103
thoracic cat 52

thoracic twist 68
time for training 14
tipping lunge 64
training 92–9
　goals 108–9
　indoor 162–7
　lactate threshold (LTHR) 109–10
　mass-participation rides 178–9
　Olympic 108, 109
　programmes 113–15
　progressing and plateauing 111
　tapering 111, 113
training camps 98–9

triangle 68
tyres 20–1, 25

V

vitamin D 127, 150
VO_2 max 12, 14

The W 70
wall presses 29
weights 28, 36–8
wheels 20
winter training 94